THE ESSENCE OF
TAI CHI CHI KUNG
-Health and Martial Arts-

Cover:
   Use the Root of Tai Chi to Reach the Goal of Wu Chi.

Dr. YANG JWING-MING

DISCLAIMER

The author(s) and publisher of this material are **NOT RESPON-SIBLE** in any manner whatsoever for any injury which may occur through reading or following the instructions in this material.

The activities, physical and otherwise, described in this material may be too strenuous or dangerous for some people, and the reader(s) should consult a physician before engaging in them.

YMAA PUBLICATION CENTER
YANG'S MARTIAL ARTS ASSOCIATION (YMAA)
38 HYDE PARK AVENUE
JAMAICA PLAIN, MASSACHUSETTS 02130

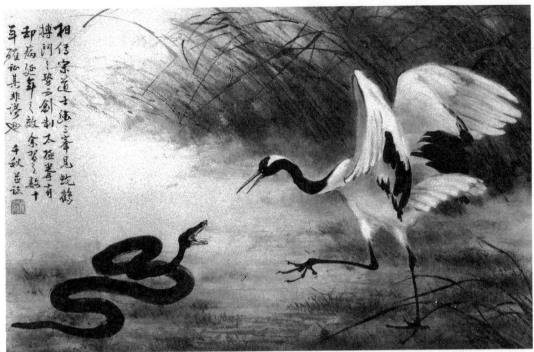

Painted by Chow Chian-Chiu

Text:

It is said that the Song Taoist Chang San-Feng, after he saw the way a crane and a snake fought, created Tai Chi Chuan, which is effective for sickness prevention and longevity. I have practiced Tai Chi for many decades and have verified this saying.

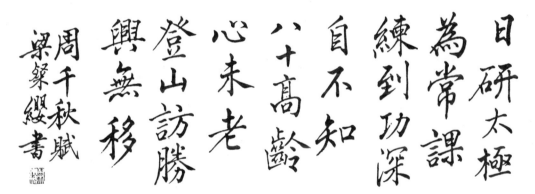

I study Tai Chi everyday as a regular lesson

I have achieved the deep Kung Fu, though I didn't realize it

At the great age of eighty, my heart is not yet old

Climbing mountains and visiting well-known scenes have never lost my interest

Poetry by Chow Chian-Chiu
Calligraphy by Leung Chen-Ying
Translation by Dr. Yang Jwing-Ming

ACKNOWLEDGEMENT

Thanks to A. Reza Farman-Farmaian for the photography, Wen-Ching Wu for the drawings, Michael Wiederhold for the typesetting, and John R. Redmond for the cover drawing. Thanks also to David Ripianzi, Roger Whidden Jr., James O'Leary, Jr., and many other YMAA members for proofing the manuscript and for contributing many valuable suggestions and discussions. Special thanks to Alan Dougall for his editing. And a very special thanks to the artists Chow Chian-Chiu and Chow Leung Chen-Ying for their beautiful painting and calligraphy on the front page of this book.

ABOUT THE AUTHOR

Dr. Yang was born in Taiwan, Republic of China, in 1946. He started his Kung Fu/Wushu training at the age of fifteen under the Shaolin White Crane (Pai Huo) master Cheng Gin-Gsao. At sixteen Dr. Yang began the study of Tai Chi Chuan (Yang Style) under Master Kao Tao.

Dr. Yang practiced Tai Chi with Master Kao for nearly three years. During this period, he learned the Yang style barehand form, Tai Chi breathing, and Chi circulation exercises. This was the beginning of Dr. Yang's involvement with Chi Kung. Through his Tai Chi practice, Dr. Yang gained an understanding of the fundamentals of Chi Kung training, especially the sitting practice for small circulation (Sheau Jou Tian).

When Dr. Yang was eighteen, he entered Tamkang College in Taipei Hsien to study Physics. While there, he began the study of Shaolin Long Fist (Chang Chuan) with Master Li Mao-Ching. At the same time, he advanced his Tai Chi training with Master Li. Later, he also practiced and studied together with his classmate Mr. Wilson Chen, who was learning Tai Chi Chuan with one of the most famous Tai Chi masters in Taipei, Master Chang Shyang-Shan. From these efforts, and through the continued studying of Tai Chi and Chi Kung books, Dr. Yang and Mr. Chen were able to greatly increase their understanding of the internal arts.

In 1971 Dr. Yang completed his M.S. degree in Physics at the National Taiwan University, and then served in the Chinese Air Force. After his honorable discharge, he returned to Tamkang College to teach Physics and resume study under Master Li Mao-Ching.

In 1974, Dr. Yang came to the United States to study Mechanical Engineering at Purdue University. Dr. Yang founded the Purdue University Chinese Kung Fu Research Club and also taught college credited courses in Tai Chi Chuan. In 1978 he was awarded a Ph.D. in Mechanical Engineering.

In 1980, Dr. Yang went to Houston and worked for Texas Instruments. While in Houston he founded Yang's Shaolin Kung Fu Academy, which was taken over by his student, Mr. Jeffery Bolt, after he moved to Boston in 1982. While Dr. Yang was continuing his engineering career, he also founded Yang's Martial Arts Academy (YMAA) on October 1, 1982 in Boston.

In January of 1984 he gave up his engineering career to devote more time to research, writing, and teaching in Boston. Dr. Yang has also travelled to France, Italy, England, Poland, West Germany, and Switzerland to share his knowledge through lectures and seminars. Dr. Yang has written fourteen books and published six videotapes. The organization has continued to expand, and, as of July 1st 1989, YMAA has become just one division of Yang's Oriental Arts Association, Inc. (YOAA, Inc).

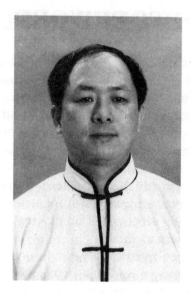

Dr. Yang Jwing-Ming

FOREWORD

Since Chinese acupuncture was introduced to the Western world, the idea of Chi and its circulation in the human body has gradually become recognized and accepted by Western doctors and the general public. More and more, people in this country are turning to acupuncture treatments or trying Chi Kung, and as they tell their friends of their good experiences, the reputation of these Oriental arts increases.

Practicing Chi Kung (which is the science of working with Chi, the energy within the body) can not only maintain your health and mental balance, but can also cure a number of illnesses without the use of any drugs. Chi Kung uses either still or moving meditation to increase and regulate the Chi circulation.

When you practice regularly, your mind will gradually become calm and peaceful, and your whole being will start to feel more balanced. However, the most important result that will come from the regular practice of Chi Kung is your discovery of the inner world of your body's energy. Through sensing and feeling, and examining your inner experiences, you will start to understand yourself not only physically but also mentally. This science of internal sensing, which the Chinese have been studying for several thousand years, has usually been totally ignored by the Western world. However, in today's busy and confusing society, this training is especially important. With the mental peace and calmness that Chi Kung can provide, you will be better able to relax and enjoy your daily work, and perhaps even find real happiness.

I believe that it is very important for the Western world to learn, study, research, and develop this scientific internal art immediately and on a wide scale. I believe that it can be very effective in helping people, especially young people, to cope with the confusing and frightening challenges of life. The general practice of Chi Kung would reduce the mental pressure in our society, help those who are unbalanced, and perhaps even lower the crime rate. Chi Kung balances the internal energy and can heal many illnesses. Older people especially will find that it will maintain their health and even slow the aging process. In addition, Chi Kung will help older people to conquer depression, and to find peace, calmness, and real happiness.

I am confident that people in the Western world will realize, as have millions of Chinese, that Chi Kung practice will give them a new outlook on life, and that it will turn out to be a key to solving many of today's problems.

For these reasons, I have been actively studying, researching, and publishing what I have learned. However, after a few years of effort, I feel that what I have accomplished is too slow and shallow. The reason for this is simply that YMAA is young and lacks the financial foundation to handle such a large and important job. I and the few people like me who are struggling to spread the word about Chi Kung cannot do it well enough by ourselves. We need to get more people involved, but we especially need to have universities and established medical organizations get involved in the research.

Since I came to United States in 1974, I have dreamed of introducing the traditional Chinese Chi Kung treasures to Western society. It is only in the last few years that this dream has gradually begun to be realized. In 1982 YMAA was organized, and in 1989 YOAA, Inc. was established. YMAA is publishing two series of Chi Kung books. The first series is for the Chi Kung beginner, and the second series is in-depth books for more experienced Chi Kung practitioners. The first book and videotape of the introductory series was "The Eight Pieces of Brocade." This book, "The Essence of Tai Chi Chi Kung," is the second of the introductory series. It will include an introduction to Chi Kung theory, which cannot be provided effectively in the videotape that is published in conjunction with this book.

If this book does not satisfy your curiosity about Chi Kung, you are invited to investigate the in-depth Chi Kung series. That series includes:

1. *THE ROOT OF CHINESE CHI KUNG* - The Secrets of Chi Kung Training (1989)
2. *MUSCLE/TENDON CHANGING AND MARROW/BRAIN WASHING CHI KUNG* - The Secret of Youth (Yi Gin Ching and Shii Soei Ching)(1989)
3. *CHI KUNG MASSAGE* - Chi Kung Tuei Na and Cavity Press for Healing (Chi Kung Ann Mo and Chi Kung Dien Shiuh)(to be published)
4. *CHI KUNG AND HEALTH* - For Healing and Maintaining Health (to be published)
5. *CHI KUNG AND MARTIAL ARTS* - The Key to Advanced Martial Arts Skill (Shaolin, Wuudang, Ermei, and others)(to be published)
6. *BUDDHIST CHI KUNG* - Charn, The Root of Zen (to be published)
7. *TAOIST CHI KUNG* (Dan Diing Tao Kung)(to be published)
8. *TIBETAN CHI KUNG* (Mih Tzong Shen Kung)(to be published)

The first volume, "The Root of Chinese Chi Kung" introduces the historical background and the different categories of Chi Kung, Chi

Kung theory and principles, and the keys to Chi Kung training. It provides a map of the world of Chi Kung. It is recommended that "The Root of Chinese Chi Kung" be read before any of the others. The second volume, "Muscle/Tendon Changing and Marrow/Brain Washing Chi Kung," introduces the general concepts of the two arts, discusses both theory and training principles of Muscle/Tendon Changing Chi Kung and of Marrow/Brain Washing Chi Kung.

To conclude, I would like to point out one thing to those of you who are sincerely interested in studying and researching this "new" science. If you start now, future generations will view you as a pioneer of the scientific investigation of Chi Kung. In addition to improving your own health, you will share the credit for raising our understanding of life as well as increasing the store of happiness in this world.

PREFACE

In the last twenty years, the Chinese concept of "Chi" has gradually come to be understood by the Western public and accepted by modern medical society. It is now believed that Chi is the "bioelectricity" circulating in the human body. It is only in the last twenty years that the field of bioelectricity has gradually opened up in modern science. Because of the interest in this new field of study, and also because of the more open communication with Chinese culture, this field will probably bloom in the next twenty years. The most obvious indications of this are the widespread acceptance of acupuncture treatment for illness and the popularity of Chi Kung and Tai Chi Chuan.

Surprisingly, the main reason for the popularity of Tai Chi Chuan is not its martial potential, but rather its ability to improve health. Although it is a martial art, Tai Chi Chuan brings the practitioner to a high level of body relaxation, calmness, and peace of mind. Most important of all, it improves the internal Chi circulation, which is the key to maintaining health and curing many illnesses.

Unlike other internal martial styles such as Hsing Yi, Ba Kua, and Liu Ho Ba Fa, the beginning training of Tai Chi Chuan is completely relaxed and the use of the muscles is reduced to a minimum. Because of this, it can be practiced by people of all ages. According to my personal teaching experience, a large percentage of people beginning Tai Chi are ill or elderly. Especially in China, Tai Chi is well known for its ability to improve or even cure many illnesses, notably problems of the stomach, lungs, heart, kidneys, high blood pressure, arthritis, mental disorders, and many others. Once you understand the principles of Chi Kung and Tai Chi training theory, you will be able to understand how this can be.

Although Tai Chi Chuan can give you a relaxed body and a calm mind, the most important benefit you can gain is a higher level of understanding of life and nature. Tai Chi leads you to the path by which you can use energy to communicate with nature. This is the path to both physical health and mental or spiritual health. Once you have achieved this, how can you wonder about or be unsure of the meaning of life?

The Chi Kung sets used in Tai Chi Chuan are simple exercises which give you a feeling for your Chi, and start you on the road to understanding how to work with your Chi. It does not just improve your Chi circulation, it is the key to the successful practice of Tai Chi Chuan for either health or martial purposes. In fact, there is not much difference between Tai Chi Chi Kung and Tai Chi Chuan itself. All of the requirements for correct practice are exactly the same for both of them. The only difference is that the Chi Kung forms are much simpler than the Tai Chi Chuan movements. This allows the practitioner to concentrate all of his effort on improving his ability to feel inside his body. Some of the forms in the Chi Kung sets are actually simplified movements adapted from the Tai Chi Chuan sequence.

There are a number of different styles of Tai Chi Chuan, each with their own Chi Kung sets. In this book I will introduce the ones which have been passed down to me from my masters. The first chapter will review the historical background of Chi Kung and Tai Chi Chuan, and introduce the general theoretical and training concepts of Chi Kung. The second chapter will discuss the root or essence of the Tai Chi training theory: Yin and Yang. Finally, the third chapter will introduce the Tai Chi Chi Kung exercises.

CONTENTS

ACKNOWLEDGEMENTS
ABOUT THE AUTHOR
FOREWORD
PREFACE

Chapter 1
General Introduction

1-1. Introduction

Chi Kung, the study of the energy in the universe, is one of the greatest cultural achievements which China has contributed to the human race. It was through the study of Chi that the balance between the Yin and Yang forces in the universe was understood. This understanding led to the formulation of the "Tao" (the natural way, pronounced "Dow"), which became one of the guiding principles of Chinese philosophy. Naturally, this "Tao" has been used to explain not only nature, but also mankind. The Chinese have hoped that the study of the Tao could show the way to improve one's health or even to extend one's life. This led to the development of Chinese medicine. The circulation of Chi in the body was studied, which became the field of human Chi Kung.

According to Chinese medical theory, the Chi or energy body is considered Yin, while the physical body is considered Yang. Chi cannot be seen, but it can be felt. The Yin aspect of your body is related to your thinking, soul, and spirit, while the Yang aspect executes the decisions of the Yin. Neither part can survive by itself. They must balance and coordinate with each other so that life can exist. Chi is the source of life, and the actions of the physical body are the manifestation of life. When the Yin is strong, the manifestation of Yang can also be strong. When Yin is weak or too strong, the Yin and Yang may lose balance and sickness can result. For this reason, Chinese medicine and Chi Kung are primarily concerned with how to maintain the correct balance of Yin and Yang.

According to many documents, although many other cultures have discovered the circulation of Chi, none of them have studied it as deeply as the Chinese. It was only in the last twenty years that the Western world has begun to accept the concept of Chi, equating it with the bioelectricity circulating in the human body. More and more, Western doctors are starting to recognize that abnormal or irregular Chi or bioelectric circulation is one of the main causes of physical and mental illnesses. Many Western physicians are sending patients to acupuncturists for an alternative method of treatment for certain diseases that Western medicine has difficulty treating. Some are even encouraging patients to take up Chi Kung or Tai Chi as a means of regulating blood pressure.

As a Chi Kung practitioner, you should trace back its history to see how it was developed. Understanding the past makes it possible for you to avoid repeating the mistakes that other people have made. It also helps you to develop an appreciation for the art, which is necessary in pursuing your own study.

For these reasons, we will devote the rest of this chapter to defining Chi and Chi Kung and reviewing the history of Chi Kung and Tai Chi Chuan. We will also introduce the general concepts which are critical in understanding the why and how of your Chi Kung practice. In the second chapter we will discuss the Yin and Yang of Tai Chi Chuan. This will give you an understanding of Tai Chi Chi Kung's place in Chinese Chi Kung. Finally, in the third chapter we will introduce several sets of Tai Chi Chi Kung exercises.

1-2. The Definition of Chi and Chi Kung

What is Chi?

In order to understand Chi Kung, you must first understand what Chi is. Chi is the energy or natural force which fills the universe. There are three general types of Chi. The heavens (the sky or universe) have Heaven Chi (Tian Chi), which is made up of the forces which the heavenly bodies exert on the earth, such as sunshine, moonlight, and the moon's effect on the tides. The Earth has Earth Chi (Dih Chi), which absorbs the Heaven Chi, and is influenced by it. Mankind has Human Chi (Ren Chi), which is influenced by the other two. In ancient times, the Chinese believed that it was Heaven Chi which controlled the weather, climate, and natural disasters. When this Chi or energy field loses its balance, it strives to rebalance itself. Then the wind must blow, rain must fall, even tornados and hurricanes must happen in order for the Heaven Chi to reach a new energy balance. Heaven Chi also affects Human Chi, and divination and astrology are attempts to explain this.

Under Heaven Chi is the Earth Chi. It is influenced and controlled by the Heaven Chi. For example, too much rain will force a river to flood or change its path. Without rain, the plants will die. The Chinese believe that Earth Chi is made up of lines and patterns of energy, as well as the earth's magnetic field and the heat concealed underground. These energies must also balance, otherwise disasters such as earthquakes will occur. When the Chi of the earth is balanced, plants will grow and animals will prosper. Also, each individual person, animal, and plant has its own Chi field, which always seeks to be balanced. When any individual life loses its balance, it will sicken, die, and decompose.

You must understand that all natural things, including man, grow within, and are influenced by, the natural cycles of Heaven Chi and Earth Chi. Since you are part of this nature (Tao), you must understand Heaven Chi and Earth Chi. Then you will be able to adjust yourself, when necessary, to fit more smoothly into the natural cycle, and you will learn how to protect yourself from the negative influences in nature. This is the major target of Chi Kung practice.

From this you can see that in order to have a long and healthy life, the first rule is that you must live in harmony with the cycles of nature, and avoid and prevent negative influences. The Chinese have researched nature for thousands of years. Some of the information on the patterns and cycles of nature has been recorded in books, one of which is the I Ching (Classic of Changes). This book gives the average person formulas to trace when the season will change, when it will snow, when a farmer should plow or harvest. You must remember that nature is always repeating itself. If you observe carefully, you will be able to see many of these routine patterns and cycles caused by the rebalancing of the Chi fields.

For thousands of years the Chinese have researched the interrelationships of all things in nature, especially with regard to human beings. From this experience they have created various Chi Kung exercises to help bring the body's Chi circulation into harmony with nature's cycles. This helps to avoid illnesses caused by weather or seasonal changes.

The Chinese also discovered that through Chi Kung they were able to strengthen their Chi circulation and slow down the degeneration of the body, gaining not only health but also a longer life. The realization that such things were possible greatly spurred new research.

What is Chi Kung?

You can see from the preceding discussion that Chi is energy, and it is found in the heavens, in the earth, and in every living thing. All of these different types of energy interact with each other, and can convert into each other. In China, the word "Kung" is often used instead of "Kung Fu," which means energy and time. Any study or training which requires a lot of energy and time to learn or to accomplish is called Kung Fu. The term can be applied to any special skill or study as long as it requires time, energy, and patience. Therefore, the correct definition of Chi Kung is any training or study dealing with Chi which takes a long time and a lot of effort.

Chi exists in everything, from the largest to the smallest. Since the range of Chi is so vast, the Chinese have divided it into three categories, parallel to the Three Powers (San Tsair) of Heaven, Earth, and Man. Generally speaking, Heaven Chi is the biggest and the most powerful. This Heaven Chi contains within it the Earth Chi, and within this Heaven and Earth Chi lives man, with his own Chi. You can see that Human Chi is part of Heaven Chi and Earth Chi. However, since the human beings who research Chi are mainly interested in Human Chi, the term Chi Kung is usually used to refer only to Chi training for people.

Chi Kung research should ideally include Heaven Chi, Earth Chi, and Human Chi. Understanding Heaven Chi is very difficult, however, and it was especially so in ancient times when the science was just developing. The major rules and principles relating to Heaven Chi can be found in such books as The Five Elements and Ten Stems, Celestial Stems, and the I Ching.

Many people have become proficient in the study of Earth Chi. They are called Dih Lii Shy (Geomancy Teachers) or Feng Shoei Shy (Wind Water Teachers). These experts use the accumulated body of geomantic knowledge and the I Ching to help people make important decisions such as where and how to build a house, or even where to locate a grave. This profession is still quite common in China.

The Chinese people believe that Human Chi is affected and controlled by Heaven Chi and Earth Chi, and that they in fact determine your destiny. Some people specialize in explaining these connections; they are called Suann Ming Shy (Calculate Life Teachers), or fortune tellers.

Most Chi Kung research has focused on Human Chi. Since Chi is the source of life, if you understand how Chi functions and know how to affect it correctly, you should be able to live a long and healthy life. Many different aspects of Human Chi have been researched, including acupuncture, acupressure, massage, herbal treatment, meditation, and Chi Kung exercises. The use of acupuncture, acupressure, massage, and herbal treatment to adjust Human Chi flow has become the root of Chinese medical science. Meditation and moving Chi Kung exercises are widely used by the Chinese people to improve their health or even to cure certain illnesses. Meditation and Chi Kung exercises serve an additional role in that Taoists and Buddhists use them in their spiritual pursuit of enlightenment and Buddhahood.

You can see that the study of any of the aspects of Chi should be called Chi Kung. However, since the term is usually used today only in reference to the cultivation of Human Chi, we will use it only in this narrower sense to avoid confusion.

1-3. A Brief History of Chi Kung

The history of Chinese Chi Kung can be roughly divided into four periods. We know little about the first period, which is considered to have started when the "I Ching" (Book of Changes) was introduced sometime before 1122 B.C., and to have extended until the Han dynasty (206 B.C.) when Buddhism and its meditation methods were imported from India. This infusion brought Chi Kung practice and meditation into the second period, the religious Chi Kung era. This period lasted until the Liang dynasty (502-557 A.D.), when it was discovered that Chi Kung could be used for martial purposes. This was the beginning of the third period, that of martial Chi Kung. Many different martial Chi Kung styles were created based on the theories and principles of Buddhist and Taoist Chi Kung. This period lasted until the overthrow of the Ching dynasty in 1911, when the new era started in which Chinese Chi Kung training is being mixed with Chi Kung practices from India, Japan, and many other countries.

Before the Han Dynasty (Before 206 B.C.)

The "I Ching" (Book of Changes; 1122 B.C.) was probably the first Chinese book related to Chi. It introduced the concept of the three natural energies or powers (San Tsair): Tian (Heaven), Dih (Earth), and Ren (Man). Studying the relationship of these three natural powers was the first step in the development of Chi Kung.

In 1766-1154 B.C. (the Shang dynasty), the Chinese capital was in today's An Yang in Henan province. An archaeological dig there at a late Shang dynasty burial ground called Yin Shiu discovered more than 160,000 pieces of turtle shell and animal bone which were covered with written characters. This writing, called "Jea Guu Wen" (Oracle-Bone Scripture), was the earliest evidence of the Chinese use of the written word. Most of the information recorded was of a religious nature. There was no mention of acupuncture or other medical knowledge, even though it was recorded in the Nei Ching that during the reign of the Yellow emperor (2690-2590 B.C.) Bian Shyr (Stone Probes) were already being used to adjust people's Chi circulation.

During the Jou dynasty (1122-934 B.C.), Lao Tzyy (Li Erh) mentioned certain breathing techniques in his classic "Tao Te Ching" (Classic on the Virtue of the Tao). He stressed that the way to obtain health was to "concentrate on Chi and achieve softness" (Juan Chi Jyh Rou)(*1). Later, "Shyy Gi" (Historical Record) in the Spring and Autumn and Warring States Periods (770-221 B.C.) also described more complete methods of breath training. About 300 B.C. the Taoist philosopher Juang Tzyy described the relationship between health and breathing in his book "Nan Hwa Ching." It states: "The men of old breathed clear down to their heels..." This was not a figure of speech, and confirms that a breathing method for Chi circulation was being used by some Taoists at that time.

During the Chin and Han dynasties (221 B.C.-220 A.D.) there are several medical references to Chi Kung in the literature, such as the "Nan Ching" (Classic on Disorders) by the famous doctor Bian Chiueh, which describes using breathing to increase Chi circulation. "Gin Guey Yao Liueh" (Prescriptions from the Golden Chamber) by Chang Jong-Jiing discusses the use of breathing and acupuncture to maintain good Chi flow. "Jou I Tsan Torng Chih" (A Comparative Study of the Jou (dynasty) Book of Changes) by Wey Bor-Yang explains the relationship of human beings to nature's forces and Chi. You can see that during this period almost all of the Chi Kung publications were written by scholars such as Lao Tzyy and Juang Tzyy, or medical doctors such as Bian Chiueh and Wey Bor-Yang.

(*1). 專氣致柔

From the Han Dynasty to the Beginning of the Liang Dynasty (206 B.C.-502 A.D.)

Because many Han emperors were intelligent and wise, the Han dynasty was a glorious and peaceful period. It was during the Eastern Han dynasty (c. 58 A.D.) that Buddhism was imported to China from India. The Han emperor became a sincere Buddhist, and Buddhism soon spread and became very popular. Many Buddhist meditation and Chi Kung practices, which had been used in India for thousands of years, were absorbed into the Chinese culture. The Buddhist temples taught many Chi Kung practices, especially the still meditation of Charn (Zen), which marked a new era of Chinese Chi Kung. Much of the deeper Chi Kung theory and practices which had been developed in India were brought to China. Unfortunately, since the training was directed at attaining Buddhahood, the training practices and theory were recorded in the Buddhist bibles and kept secret. For hundreds of years the religious Chi Kung training was never taught to laymen. Only in this century has it been available to the general populace.

Not long after Buddhism was imported into China, a Taoist by the name of Chang Tao-Ling combined the traditional Taoist principles with Buddhism and created a religion called Tao Jiaw. Many of the meditation methods were a combination of the principles and training methods of both sources.

Since Tibet had its own branch of Buddhism with its own training system and methods of attaining Buddhahood, Tibetan Buddhists were also invited to China to preach. In time, their practices were also absorbed.

It was in this period that the traditional Chinese Chi Kung practitioners finally had a chance to compare their arts with the religious Chi Kung practices imported mainly from India. While the scholarly and medical Chi Kung had been concerned with maintaining and improving health, the newly imported religious Chi Kung was concerned with far more. Contemporary documents and Chi Kung styles show clearly that the religious practitioners trained their Chi to a much deeper level, working with many internal functions of the body, and strove to have control of their bodies, minds, and spirits with the goal of escaping from the cycle of reincarnation.

While the Chi Kung practices and meditations were being passed down secretly within the monasteries, traditional scholars and physicians continued their Chi Kung research. During the Gin dynasty in the 3rd century A.D., a famous physician named Hwa Tor used acupuncture for anesthesia in surgery. The Taoist Jiun Chiam used the movements of animals to create the Wuu Chyn Shih (Five Animal Sports), which taught people how to increase their Chi circulation through specific movements. Also, in this period a physician named Ger Horng mentioned using the mind to lead and increase Chi in his book Baw Poh Tzyy. Sometime in the period of 420 to 581 A.D. Taur Horng-Jiing compiled the "Yeang Shenn Yan Ming Luh"

(Records of Nourishing the Body and Extending Life), which showed many Chi Kung techniques.

From the Liang Dynasty to the End of the Ching Dynasty (502-1911 A.D.)

During the Liang dynasty (502-557 A.D.) the emperor invited a Buddhist monk named Da Mo, who was once an Indian prince, to preach Buddhism in China. When the emperor decided he did not like Da Mo's Buddhist theory, the monk withdrew to the Shaolin Temple. When Da Mo arrived, he saw that the priests were weak and sickly, so he shut himself away to ponder the problem. He emerged after nine years of seclusion and wrote two classics: "Yi Gin Ching" (Muscle/-Tendon Changing Classic) and "Shii Soei Ching" (Marrow/Brain Washing Classic). The Muscle/Tendon Changing Classic taught the priests how to gain health and change their physical bodies from weak to strong. The Marrow/Brain Washing Classic taught the priests how to use Chi to clean the bone marrow and strengthen the blood and immune systems, as well as how to energize the brain and attain enlightenment. Because the Marrow/Brain Washing Classic was harder to understand and practice, the training methods were passed down secretly to only a very few disciples in each generation.

After the priests practiced the Muscle/Tendon Changing exercises, they found that not only did they improve their health, but they also greatly increased their strength. When this training was integrated into the martial arts forms, it increased the effectiveness of their techniques. In addition to this martial Chi Kung training, the Shaolin priests also created five animal styles of Kung Fu which imitated the way different animals fight. The animals imitated were the tiger, leopard, dragon, snake, and crane.

Outside of the monastery, the development of Chi Kung continued during the Swei and Tarng dynasties (581-907 A.D.). Chaur Yuan-Fang compiled the "Ju Bing Yuan Hou Luenn" (Thesis on the Origins and Symptoms of Various Diseases), which is a veritable encyclopedia of Chi Kung methods listing 260 different ways of increasing the Chi flow. The "Chian Gin Fang" (Thousand Gold Prescriptions) by Suen Sy-Meau described the method of leading Chi, and also described the use of the Six Sounds. The use of the Six Sounds to regulate Chi in the internal organs had already been used by the Buddhists and Taoists for some time. Suen Sy-Meau also introduced a massage system called Lao Tzyy's 49 Massage Techniques. "Wai Tai Mih Yao" (The Extra Important Secret) by Wang Tour discussed the use of breathing and herbal therapies for disorders of Chi circulation.

During the Song, Gin, and Yuan dynasties (960-1368 A.D.), "Yeang Shenn Jyue" (Life Nourishing Secrets) by Chang An-Tao discussed several Chi Kung practices. "Ru Men Shyh Shyh" (The Confucian Point of View) by Chang Tzyy-Her describes the use of Chi Kung to cure external injuries such as cuts and sprains. "Lan Shyh Mih Tsarng" (Secret Library of the Orchid Room) by Li Guoo describes using Chi Kung and herbal remedies for internal disorders. "Ger Jyh Yu Luenn" (A Further Thesis of Complete Study) by Ju Dan-Shi provided a theoretical explanation for the use of Chi Kung in curing disease.

During the Song dynasty (960-1279 A.D.), Chang San-Feng is believed to have created Tai Chi Chuan. Tai Chi followed a different approach in its use of Chi Kung than did Shaolin. While Shaolin emphasized Wai Dan (External Elixir) Chi Kung exercises, Tai Chi emphasized Nei Dan (Internal Elixir) Chi Kung training.

In 1026 A.D. the famous brass man of acupuncture was designed and built by Dr. Wang Wei-Yi. Before this time, although there were many publications which discussed acupuncture theory, principles, and treatment techniques, there were many disagreements among them, and many points which were unclear. When Dr. Wang built his brass man, he also wrote a book called "Torng Ren Yu Shiuh Jen Jeou Twu" (Illustration of the Brass Man Acupuncture and Moxibustion). He explained the relationship of the 12 organs and the 12 Chi channels, clarified many of the points of confusion, and, for the first time, systematically organized acupuncture theory and principles.

In 1034 A.D. Dr. Wang used acupuncture to cure the emperor Ren Tzong. With the support of the emperor, acupuncture flourished. In order to encourage acupuncture medical research, the emperor built a temple to Bian Chiueh, who wrote the Nan Ching, and worshiped him as the ancestor of acupuncture. Acupuncture technology developed so much that even the Gin race in the North requested the brass man and other acupuncture technology as a condition for peace. Between 1102 to 1106 A.D. Dr. Wang dissected the bodies of prisoners and added more information to the Nan Ching. His work contributed greatly to the advancement of Chi Kung and Chinese medicine by giving a clear and systematic idea of the circulation of Chi in the human body.

Later, in the Southern Song dynasty (1127-1279 A.D.), Marshal Yeuh Fei was credited with creating several internal Chi Kung exercises and martial arts. It is said that he created the Eight Pieces of Brocade to improve the health of his soldiers. He is also known as the creator of the internal martial style Hsing Yi. Eagle style martial artists also claim that Yeuh Fei was the creator of their style.

From then until the end of the Ching dynasty (1911 A.D.), many other Chi Kung styles were founded. The well known ones include Hwu Buh Kung (Tiger Step Kung), Shyr Er Juang (Twelve Postures) and Jiaw Huah Kung (Beggar Kung). Also in this period, many documents related to Chi Kung were published, such as "Bao Shenn Mih Yao" (The Secret Important Document of Body Protection) by Tsaur Yuan-Bair, which described moving and stationary Chi Kung practices; and "Yeang Shenn Fu Yeu" (Brief Introduction to Nourishing the Body) by Chen Jih-Ru, about the three treasures: Jieng (Essence), Chi (Internal Energy), and Shen (Spirit). Also, "Yi Fang Jyi Jieh" (The Total Introduction to Medical Prescriptions) by Uang Fann-An reviewed and summarized the previously published materials; and

"Nei Kung Twu Shwo" (Illustrated Explanation of Nei Kung) by Wang Tzuu-Yuan presented the Twelve Pieces of Brocade and explained the idea of combining both moving and stationary Chi Kung.

In the late Ming dynasty (around 1640 A.D.), a martial Chi Kung style, Huoo Long Kung (Fire Dragon Kung) was created by the Tai Yang martial stylists. The well known internal martial art style Ba Kua Chang (Eight Trigrams Palm) is believed to have been created by Doong Hae-Chuan late in the Ching dynasty (1644-1911 A.D.). This style is now gaining in popularity throughout the world.

During the Ching dynasty, Tibetan meditation and martial techniques became widespread in China for the first time. This was due to the encouragement and interest of the Manchurian Emperors in the royal palace, as well as others of high rank in society.

From the End of Ching Dynasty to the Present

Before 1911 A.D., Chinese society was still very conservative and old fashioned. Even though China had been expanding its contact with the outside world for the previous hundred years, the outside world had little influence beyond the coastal regions. With the overthrow of the Ching dynasty in 1911 and the founding of the Chinese Republic, the nation started changing as never before. Since this time Chi Kung practice has entered a new era. Because of the ease of communication in the modern world, Western culture is having a great influence on the Orient. Many Chinese have opened their minds and changed their traditional ideas, especially in Taiwan and Hong Kong. Various Chi Kung styles are now being taught openly, and many formerly secret documents have been published. Modern methods of communication have opened up Chi Kung to a much wider audience than ever before, and people now have the chance to study and understand many different styles. In addition, people are now able to compare Chinese Chi Kung to similar arts from other countries such as India, Japan, Korea, and the Middle East.

I believe that in the near future Chi Kung will be considered the most exciting and challenging field of research. It is an ancient science just waiting to be investigated with the help of the new technologies now being developed at an almost explosive rate. Anything we can do to speed up this research will greatly help humanity to understand and improve itself.

1-4. Categories of Chi Kung

Generally speaking, all Chi Kung practices can be divided according to their training theory and methods into two general categories: Wai Dan (External Elixir) and Nei Dan (Internal Elixir). Understanding the differences between them will give you an overview of most Chinese Chi Kung practices.

1. Wai Dan (External Elixir)

"Wai" means "external or outside," and "Dan" means "elixir." External here means the limbs, as opposed to the torso, which includes all of the vital organs. Elixir is a hypothetical, life-prolong-ing substance for which Chinese Taoists have been searching for millennia. They originally thought that the elixir was something physical which could be prepared from herbs or chemicals purified in a furnace. After thousands of years of study and experimentation, they found that the elixir is in the body. In other words, if you want to prolong your life, you must find the elixir in your body, and then learn to protect and nourish it.

In Wai Dan Chi Kung practice, you concentrate your attention on your limbs. As you exercise, the Chi builds up in your arms and legs. When the Chi potential in your limbs builds to a high enough level, the Chi will flow through the channels, clearing any obstructions and nourishing the organs. This is the main reason that a person who works out, or has a physical job, is generally healthier than someone who sits around all day.

2. Nei Dan (Internal Elixir)

Nei means internal and Dan means elixir. Thus, Nei Dan means to build the elixir internally. Here, internally means in the body instead of in the limbs. Whereas in Wai Dan the Chi is built up in the limbs and then moved into the body, Nei Dan exercises build up Chi in the body and lead it out to the limbs.

Generally speaking, Nei Dan theory is deeper than Wai Dan theory, and it is more difficult to understand and practice. Traditionally, most of the Nei Dan Chi Kung practices have been passed down more secretly than those of the Wai Dan. This is especially true of the highest levels of Nei Dan, such as Marrow/Brain Washing, which were passed down to only a few trusted disciples.

We can also classify Chi Kung into four major categories according to the purpose or final goal of the training: 1. maintaining health; 2. curing sickness; 3. martial skill; and 4. enlightenment or Buddhahood. This is only a rough breakdown, however, since almost every style of Chi Kung serves more than one of the above purposes. For example, although martial Chi Kung focuses on increasing fighting effectiveness, it can also improve your health. The Taoist Chi Kung aims for longevity and enlightenment, but to reach this goal you need to be in good health and know how to cure sickness. Because of this multi-purpose aspect of the categories, it will be simpler to discuss their backgrounds rather than the goals of their training. Knowing the history and basic principles of each category will help you to understand their Chi Kung more clearly.

1. Scholar Chi Kung - for Maintaining Health

In China before the Han dynasty, there were two major schools of scholarship. One of them was created by Confucius (551-479 B.C.) during the Spring and Autumn Period, and the scholars who practice his philosophy are commonly called Confucians. Later, his philosophy was popularized and enlarged by Mencius (372-289 B.C.) in the Warring States Period. The people who practice this are called Ru Jia (Confucianists). The key words to their basic philosophy are Loyalty,

Filial Piety, Humanity, Kindness, Trust, Justice, Harmony, and Peace. Humanity and human feelings are the main subjects of study. Ru Jia philosophy has become the center of much of Chinese culture.

The second major school of scholarship was called Tao Jia (Taoism) and was created by Lao Tzyy in the 6th century B.C. Lao Tzyy is considered to be the author of a book called the "Tao Te Ching" (Classic on the Virtue of the Tao) which described human morality. Later, in the Warring States Period, his follower Juang Jou wrote a book called "Juang Tzyy," which led to the forming of another strong branch of Taoism. Before the Han dynasty, Taoism was considered a branch of scholarship. However, in the Han dynasty traditional Taoism was combined with the Buddhism imported from India, and it began gradually to be treated as a religion. Therefore, the Taoism before the Han dynasty should be considered scholarly Taoism rather than religious.

With regard to their contribution to Chi Kung, both schools of scholarship emphasized maintaining health and preventing disease. They believed that many illnesses are caused by mental and emotional excesses. When a person's mind is not calm, balanced, and peaceful, the organs will not function normally. For example, depression can cause stomach ulcers and indigestion. Anger will cause the liver to malfunction. Sadness will cause stagnation and tightness in the lungs, and fear can disturb the normal functioning of the kidneys and bladder. They realized that if you want to avoid illness, you must learn to balance and relax your thoughts and emotions. This is called "regulating the mind."

Therefore, the scholars emphasized gaining a peaceful mind through meditation. In their still meditation, the main part of the training is getting rid of thoughts so that the mind is clear and calm. When you become calm, the flow of thoughts and emotions slows down, and you feel mentally and emotionally neutral. This kind of meditation can be thought of as practicing emotional self-control. When you are in this "no thought" state, you become very relaxed, and can even relax deep down into your internal organs. When your body is this relaxed, your Chi will naturally flow smoothly and strongly. This kind of still meditation was very common in ancient Chinese scholarly society.

In order to reach the goal of a calm and peaceful mind, their training focused on regulating the mind, body, and breath. They believed that as long as these three things were regulated, the Chi flow would be smooth and sickness would not occur. This is why the Chi training of the scholars is called "Shiou Chi," which means "cultivating Chi." Shiou in Chinese means to regulate, to cultivate, or to repair. It means to maintain in good condition. This is very different from the Taoist Chi training after the Han dynasty which was called "Liann Chi," which is translated "train Chi." Liann means to drill or to practice to make stronger.

Many of the Chi Kung documents written by the Confucians and Taoists were limited to the maintenance of health. The scholar's attitude in Chi Kung was to follow his natural destiny and maintain his health. This philosophy is quite different from that of the Taoists after the Han dynasty, who denied that one's destiny could not be changed. They believed that it is possible to train your Chi to make it stronger, and to extend your life. It is said in scholarly society: "Ren Shenn Chii Shyr Guu Lai Shi,"(*2) which means "in human life seventy is rare." You should understand that few of the common people in ancient times lived past seventy because of the lack of good food and modern medical technology. It is also said: "An Tian Leh Ming,"(*3) which means "peace with heaven and delight in your destiny"; and "Shiou Shenn Shy Ming," (*4) which means "cultivate the body and await destiny." Compare this with the philosophy of the later Taoists, who said: "Yi Bae Er Shyr Wey Jy Yeau,"(*5) which means "one hundred and twenty means dying young." They believed and have proven that human life can be lengthened and destiny can be resisted and overcome.

Confucianism and Taoism were the two major schools of scholarship in China, but there were many other schools which were also more or less involved in Chi Kung exercises. We will not discuss them here because there is only a limited number of Chi Kung documents from these schools.

2.   Medical Chi Kung - for Healing

In ancient Chinese society, most emperors respected the scholars and were affected by their philosophy. Doctors were not regarded highly because they made their diagnosis by touching the patient's body, which was considered characteristic of the lower classes in society. Although the doctors developed a profound and successful medical science, they were commonly looked down on. However, they continued to work hard and study, and quietly passed down the results of their research to following generations.

Of all the groups studying Chi Kung in China, the doctors have been at it the longest. Since the discovery of Chi circulation in the human body about four thousand years ago, the Chinese doctors have devoted a major portion of their efforts to studying the behavior of Chi. Their efforts resulted in acupuncture, acupressure or Cavity Press massage, and herbal treatment.

In addition, many Chinese doctors used their medical knowledge to create different sets of Chi Kung exercises either for maintaining health or for curing specific illnesses. Chinese medical doctors believed that doing only sitting or still meditation to regulate the body, mind, and breathing as the scholars did was not enough to cure sickness. They believed that in order to increase the Chi circulation, you must move. Although a calm and peaceful mind was important for health, exercising the body was more important. They learned through their

---

(*2). 人生七十古來稀
(*3). 安天樂命
(*4). 修身俟命
(*5). 一百二十謂之夭

medical practice that people who exercised properly got sick less often, and their bodies degenerated less quickly than was the case with people who just sat around. They also realized that specific body movements could increase the Chi circulation in specific organs. They reasoned from this that these exercises could also be used to treat specific illnesses and to restore the normal functioning of these organs.

Some of these movements are similar to the way in which certain animals move. It is clear that in order for an animal to survive in the wild, it must have an instinct for how to protect its body. Part of this instinct is concerned with how to build up its Chi, and how to keep its Chi from being lost. We humans have lost many of these instincts over the years that we have been separating ourselves from nature.

Many doctors developed Chi Kung exercises which were modeled after animal movements to maintain health and cure sickness. A typical, well known set of such exercises is "Wuu Chyn Shih" (Five Animal Sports) created by Dr. Jiun Chiam. Another famous set based on similar principles is called "Ba Duann Gin" (The Eight Pieces of Brocade). It was created by Marshal Yeuh Fei who, interestingly enough, was a soldier rather than a doctor.

In addition, using their medical knowledge of Chi circulation, Chinese doctors researched until they found which movements could help cure particular illnesses and health problems. Not surprisingly, many of these movements were not unlike the ones used to maintain health, since many illnesses are caused by unbalanced Chi. When an imbalance continues for a long period of time, the organs will be affected, and may be physically damaged. It is just like running a machine without supplying the proper electrical current - over time, the machine will be damaged. Chinese doctors believe that before physical damage to an organ shows up in a patient's body, there is first an abnormality in the Chi balance and circulation. **ABNORMAL CHI CIRCULATION IS THE VERY BEGINNING OF ILLNESS AND PHYSICAL ORGAN DAMAGE**. When Chi is too positive (Yang) or too negative (Yin) in a specific organ's Chi channel, your physical organ is beginning to suffer damage. If you do not correct the Chi circulation, that organ will malfunction or degenerate. The best way to heal someone is to adjust and balance the Chi even before there is any physical problem. Therefore, correcting or increasing the normal Chi circulation is the major goal of acupuncture or acupressure treatments. Herbs and special diets are also considered important treatments in regulating the Chi in the body.

As long as the illness is limited to the level of Chi stagnation and there is no physical organ damage, the Chi Kung exercises used for maintaining health can be used to readjust the Chi circulation and treat the problem. However, if the sickness is already so serious that the physical organs have started to fail, then the situation has become critical and a specific treatment is necessary. The treatment can be acupuncture, herbs, or even an operation, as well as specific

Chi Kung exercises designed to speed up the healing or even to cure the sickness. For example, ulcers and asthma can often be cured or helped by some simple exercises. Recently in both mainland China and Taiwan, certain Chi Kung exercises have been shown to be effective in treating certain kinds of cancer.(*6)

Over the thousands of years of observing nature and themselves, some Chi Kung practitioners went even deeper. They realized that the body's Chi circulation changes with the seasons, and that it is a good idea to help the body out during these periodic adjustments. They noticed also that in each season different organs have characteristic problems. For example, in the beginning of Fall the lungs have to adapt to the colder air that you are breathing. While this adjustment is going on, the lungs are susceptible to disturbance, so your lungs may feel uncomfortable and you may catch colds easily. Your digestive system is also affected during seasonal changes. Your appetite may increase, or you may have diarrhea. When the temperature goes down, your kidneys and bladder will start to give you trouble. For example, because the kidneys are stressed, you may feel pain in the back. Focusing on these seasonal Chi disorders, the meditators created a set of movements which can be used to speed up the body's adjustment. These Chi Kung exercises will be introduced in a later volume.

In addition to Marshal Yeuh Fei, many people who were not doctors also created sets of medical Chi Kung. These sets were probably originally created to maintain health, and later were also used for curing sickness.

3.   Martial Chi Kung - for Fighting

Chinese martial Chi Kung was probably not developed until Da Mo wrote the Muscle/Tendon Changing Classic in the Shaolin Temple during the Liang dynasty (502-557 A.D.). When Shaolin monks trained Da Mo's Muscle/Tendon Changing Chi Kung, they found that they could not only improve their health but also greatly increase the power of their martial techniques. Since then, many martial styles have developed Chi Kung sets to increase their effectiveness. In addition, many martial styles have been created based on Chi Kung theory. Martial artists have played a major role in Chinese Chi Kung society.

When Chi Kung theory was first applied to the martial arts, it was used to increase the power and efficiency of the muscles. The theory is very simple - the mind (Yi) is used to lead Chi to the muscles to energize them so that they function more efficiently. The average person generally uses his muscles at under 40% maximum efficiency.

(*6). There are many reports in popular and professional literature of using Chi Kung to help or even cure many illnesses, including cancer. Many cases have been discussed in the Chinese Chi Kung journals. One book which describes the use of Chi Kung to cure cancer is New Chi Kung for Preventing and Curing Cancer (新氣功防治癌症), by Yeh Ming, Chinese Yoga Publications, Taiwan, 1986.

If one can train his concentration and use his strong Yi (the mind generated from clear thinking) to lead Chi to the muscles effectively, he will be able to energize the muscles to a higher level and, therefore, increase his fighting effectiveness.

As acupuncture theory became better understood, fighting techniques were able to reach even more advanced levels. Martial artists learned to attack specific areas, such as vital acupuncture cavities, to disturb the enemy's Chi flow and create imbalances which caused injury or even death. In order to do this, the practitioner must understand the route and timing of the Chi circulation in the human body. He also has to train so that he can strike the cavities accurately and to the correct depth. These cavity strike techniques are called "Dien Shiuh" (Pointing Cavities) or "Dim Mak" (Pointing Vessels).

Most of the martial Chi Kung practices help to improve the practitioner's health. However, there are other martial Chi Kung practices which, although they build up some special skill which is useful for fighting, also damage the practitioner's health. An example of this is Iron Sand Palm. Although this training can build up amazing destructive power, it can also harm your hands and affect the Chi circulation in the hands and the internal organs.

Since the 6th century, many martial styles have been created which were based on Chi Kung theory. They can be roughly divided into external and internal styles.

The external styles emphasize building Chi in the limbs to coordinate with the physical martial techniques. They follow the theory of Wai Dan (External Elixir) Chi Kung, which usually generates Chi in the limbs through special exercises. The concentrated mind is used during the exercises to energize the Chi. This increases muscular strength significantly, and therefore increases the effectiveness of the martial techniques. Chi Kung can also be used to train the body to resist punches and kicks. In this training, Chi is led to energize the skin and the muscles, enabling them to resist a blow without injury. This training is commonly called "Iron Shirt" (Tiea Bu Shan) or "Golden Bell Cover" (Gin Jong Jaw). The martial styles which use Wai Dan Chi Kung training are normally called external styles (Wai Kung) or hard styles (Ying Kung). Shaolin Kung Fu is a typical example of a style which uses Wai Dan martial Chi Kung.

Although Wai Dan Chi Kung can help the martial artist increase his power, there is a disadvantage. Because Wai Dan Chi Kung emphasizes training the external muscles, it can cause over-development. This can cause a problem called "energy dispersion" (Sann Kung) when the practitioner gets older. In order to remedy this, when an external martial artist reaches a high level of external Chi Kung training he will start training internal Chi Kung, which specializes in curing the energy dispersion problem. That is why it is said "Shaolin Kung Fu from external to internal."

Internal Martial Chi Kung is based on the theory of Nei Dan (Internal Elixir). In this method, Chi is generated in the body instead of the limbs, and this Chi is then led to the limbs to increase power. In order to lead Chi to the limbs, the techniques must be soft and muscle usage must be kept to a minimum. The training and theory of Nei Dan martial Chi Kung is much more difficult than those of Wai Dan martial Chi Kung. Interested readers should refer to the author's book: "Advanced Yang Style Tai Chi Chuan - Tai Chi Theory and Tai Chi Jing."

Several internal martial styles were created in the Wuudang and Ermei Mountains. Popular styles are Tai Chi Chuan, Ba Kua, Liu Ho Ba Fa, and Hsing Yi. However, you should understand that even the internal martial styles, which are commonly called soft styles, must on some occasions use muscular strength while fighting. Therefore, once an internal martial artist has achieved a degree of competence in internal Chi Kung, he or she should also learn how to use harder, more external techniques. That is why it is said: "the internal styles are from soft to hard."

In the last fifty years, some of the Tai Chi Chi Kung or Tai Chi Chuan practitioners have developed training which is mainly for health, and is called "Wu Chi Chi Kung," which means "no extremities Chi Kung." Wu Chi is the state of neutrality which precedes Tai Chi, which is the state of complimentary opposites. When there are thoughts and feelings in your mind, there is Yin and Yang, but if you can still your mind you can return to the emptiness of Wu Chi. When you achieve this state your mind is centered and clear and your body relaxed, and your Chi is able to flow naturally and smoothly and reach the proper balance by itself. Wu Chi Chi Kung has become very popular in many parts of China, especially Shanghai and Canton.

You can see that, although Chi Kung is widely studied in Chinese martial society, the main focus of training was originally on increasing fighting ability rather than health. Good health was considered a by-product of the training. It was not until this century that the health aspect of martial Chi Kung started receiving greater attention. This is especially true in the internal martial arts. Please refer to the future YMAA in-depth Chi Kung book series: "Chi Kung and Martial Arts."

4.   Religious Chi Kung - for Enlightenment or Buddhahood

Religious Chi Kung, though not as popular as other categories in China, is recognized as having achieved the highest accomplishments of all the Chi Kung categories. It used to be kept secret, and it is only in this century that it has been revealed to laymen.

In China, religious Chi Kung includes mainly Taoist and Buddhist Chi Kung. The main purpose of their training is striving for enlightenment, or what the Buddhists refer to as Buddhahood. They are looking for a way to lift themselves above normal human suffering, and to escape from the cycle of continual reincarnation. They believe that all human suffering is caused by the seven emotions and six desires. If you are still bound to these emotions and desires, you will reincarnate after your death. To avoid reincarnation, you must train your spirit to reach a very high stage where it is strong enough to be independent after your death. This spirit will enter the heavenly kingdom and gain eternal peace. This training is hard to do in the everyday world, so practitioners frequently flee society and move into the solitude of the mountains, where they can concentrate all of their energies on self-cultivation.

Religious Chi Kung practitioners train to strengthen their internal Chi to nourish their spirit (Shen) until this spirit is able to survive the death of the physical body. Marrow/Brain Washing Chi Kung training is necessary to reach this stage. It enables them to lead Chi to the forehead, where the spirit resides, and raise the brain to a higher energy state. This training used to be restricted to only a few priests who had reached an advanced level. Tibetan Buddhists were also involved heavily in this training. Over the last two thousand years the Tibetan Buddhists, the Chinese Buddhists, and the Taoist have followed the same principles to become the three major religious schools of Chi Kung training.

This religious striving toward enlightenment or Buddhahood is recognized as the highest and most difficult level of Chi Kung. Many Chi Kung practitioners reject the rigors of this religious striving, and practice Marrow/Brain Washing Chi Kung solely for the purpose of longevity. It was these people who eventually revealed the secrets of Marrow/Brain Washing to the outside world. If you are interested in knowing more about this training, you may refer to: "Muscle/Tendon Changing and Marrow/Brain Washing Chi Kung" by Dr. Yang.

1-5. A Brief History of Tai Chi Chuan

Chi theory and Chi Kung were not applied to the Chinese martial arts until the late Liang dynasty (502-557 A.D.). This Chi Kung can be classified as either "external" or "internal." The external styles energize the muscles in the limbs with Chi so that they can manifest their maximum strength. Naturally, such training also develops the muscles. The internal styles believe that, in order for the physical body to manifest its maximum power, the most important thing was learning how to circulate and build up the Chi. Only then could the physical body be energized effectively. Their training therefore focused on circulating and building up the Chi internally. To do this, the body must remain relaxed and, to a degree, soft. Tai Chi Chuan belongs to this internal category.

It is said that Tai Chi Chuan was created by Chang San-Feng in the Song Wei Tzong era (c. 1101 A.D.). It is also said that techniques and forms with the same basic principles were already in existence during the Liang dynasty (502-557 A.D.), and were being taught by Han Goong-Yeuh, Chen Ling-Shii, and Chen Bi. Later, in the Tarng dynasty (713-905 A.D.), it was found that Sheu Hsuan-Pin, Li Tao-Tzu, and Ien Li-Hen were teaching similar martial techniques. They were called Thirty-Seven Postures (San Shih Chi Shih), Post-Heaven Techniques (Hou Tian Faa), or Small Nine Heaven (Sheau Jeau Tian), which had seventeen postures. The accuracy of these accounts is questionable, so it is not really known when and by whom Tai Chi Chuan was created. Because there is more formal history recorded about Chang San-Feng, he has received most of the credit.

According to the historical record Nan Lei Gi Wang Jeng Nan Moo Tzu Min: "Chang San-Feng, in the Song dynasty, was a Wuudang Taoist. Wei Tzong (a Song Emperor) summoned him, but the road was blocked and he couldn't come. At night, (Wei Tzong) dreamed Emperor Yuen (the first Gin emperor) taught him martial techniques. At dawn, he killed a hundred enemies by himself."(*7) Also, recorded in the Ming history Ming Shih Fan Gi Chwan: "Chang San-Feng, from Lieu Dong Yi county. Named Chuan-Yi. Also named Jiun-Bao. San-Feng was his nickname. Because he did not keep himself neat and clean, also called Chang Lar-Tar (Sloppy Chang). He was tall and big, shaped like a turtle, and had a crane's back. Large ears and round eyes. Beard long like a spear tassel. Wears only a priest's robe winter or summer. Will eat a bushel of food, or won't eat for several days or a few months. Can travel a thousand miles. Likes to have fun with people. Behaves as if nobody is around. Used to travel to Wuudang with his disciples. Built a simple cottage and lived inside. In the 24th year of Hung Wu (around 1939), Ming Tai Tzu (the first Ming emperor) heard of his name, and set a messenger to look for him but he couldn't be found."(*8)

It was also recorded in the Ming dynasty in Ming Lan Yin Chi Shou Lei Kou: "Chang the Immortal, named Jiun-Bao, also named Chuan-Yi, nicknamed Shuan-Shuan, also called Chang Lar-Tar. In the third year of Tian Suen (1460 A.D.) he visited Emperor Ming Ying Tzong. A picture was drawn. The beard and mustache were straight, the back of the head had a tuft. Purple face and big stomach, with a bamboo hat in his hand. One the top of the picture was an inscription from the emperor honoring Chang as 'Ton Wei Sien Hua Jen Ren' (a genuine Taoist who finally discriminates and clearly understands much" (Figure 1-1)(*9). The record is suspect, because if is were true, Chang San-Feng would have been at least 500 years old at that time.

(*7). 南雷集王征南墓誌銘： " 宋之張三豐爲武當丹
士．徽宗召之．路梗不得進．夜夢元帝授之拳
法．厥明以單丁殺賊百餘． "

(*8). 明史方伎傳： " 張三豐遼東懿州人．名全一．
一名君寶．三豐其號也．以不修邊幅，又號張
邋遢，頎而偉．龜形鶴背，大耳圓目．鬚髯如
戟，寒署惟一衲蓑，所啖升斗輒盡．或數日不
食，或數月不食．一日千里．善嬉戲，旁若無
人．嘗與其徒遊武當，築草盧而居之．洪武二
十四年，太祖聞其名，遣使覓之不得． "

(*9). 明郎瑛七修類稿： " 張仙名君寶，字全一，別
號玄玄，時人又稱張邋遢．天順三年，曾來謁
帝．予見其像，鬚鬢豎立，一瞥背垂．紫面大
腹，而攜笠者．上爲錫誥之文，封爲通微顯化
真人． "

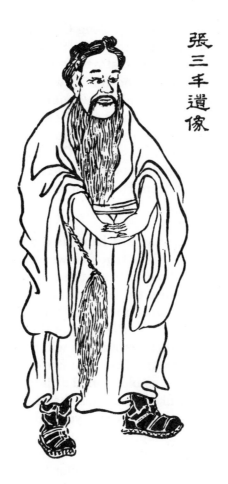

張三丰遺像

Figure 1-1.

Other records state that Chang San-Feng's techniques were learned from the Taoist Fon Yi-Yuen. Another story tells that Chang San-Feng was an ancient hermit meditator. He saw a magpie fighting a snake, had a sudden understanding, and created Tai Chi Chuan.

After Chang San-Feng, there were Wang Tzong in Shaanxi province, Chen Ton-Jou in Wen County, Chang Soun-Shi in Hai Yen, Yeh Gi-Mei in Shyh Ming, Wang Tzong-Yeuh in San You, and Chiang Fa in Hebei. The Tai Chi techniques were passed down and divided into two major styles, southern and northern. Later, Chiang Fa passed his art to the Chen family at Chen Jar Gou (Chen Village) in Hwai Ching County, Henan. Tai Chi was then passed down for fourteen generations and divided into the Old and the New Styles. The Old style was carried on by Chen Chang-Shen and the New Style was created by Chen You-Ban.

The Old Style successor Chen Chang-Shen then passed the art down to his son, Ken-Yun, and his Chen relatives, Chen Hwai-Yuen and Chen Hwa-Mei. He also passed his Tai Chi outside of his family to Yang Lu-Shann and Li Bao-Kuai, both of Hebei province. This Old Style is called Thirteen Postures Old Form (Shih San Shih Lao Jiah). Later, Yang Lu-Shann passed it down to his two sons, Yang Ban-Huo and Yang Chien-Huo. Then, Chien-Huo passed the art to his two sons, Yang Shao-Huo and Yang Chen-Fu. This branch of Tai Chi Chuan is popularly called Yang Style. Also, Wu Chun-Yu learned from Yang Ban-Huo and started a well known Wu Style.

Also, Chen You-Ban passed his New Style to Chin Ching-Pin who created Tsao Bao Style Tai Chi Chuan. Wuu Yu-Larn learned the Old Style from Yang Lu-Shann and New Style from Chen Ching-Pin, and created Wuu Style Tai Chi Chuan. Li Yi-Yu learned the Wuu Style and created Li Style Tai Chi Chuan. Heh Wei-Jinn obtained his art from Li style and created Heh Style Tai Chi Chuan. Suen Luh-Tarng learned from Heh Style and created Suen Style.

1-6. Chi Kung Theory

Many people think that Chi Kung is a difficult subject to comprehend. In some ways, this is true. However, you must understand one thing: regardless of how difficult the Chi Kung theory and practice of a particular style are, the basic theory and principles are very simple and remain the same for all of the Chi Kung styles. The basic theory and principles are the roots of the entire Chi Kung practice. If you understand these roots, you will be able to grasp the key to the practice and grow. All of the Chi Kung styles originated from these roots, but each one has blossomed differently.

In this section we will discuss these basic theories and principles. With this knowledge as a foundation, you will be able to understand not only what you should be doing, but also why you are doing it. Naturally, it is impossible to discuss all of the basic Chi Kung ideas in such a short section. However, it will offer beginners the key to open the gate into the spacious, four thousand year old garden of Chinese Chi Kung. If you wish to know more about the theory of Chi Kung, please refer to: "The Root of Chinese Chi Kung" by Dr. Yang.

Chi and Man

In order to use Chi Kung to maintain and improve your health, you must know that there is Chi in your body, and you must understand how it circulates and what you can do to insure that the circulation is smooth and strong.

You know from previous discussions that Chi is energy. It is a requirement for life. The Chi in your body cannot be seen, but it can be felt. This Chi can make your body feel too positive (too Yang) or too negative (too Yin).

Imagine that your physical body is a machine, and your Chi is the current that makes it run. Without the current the machine is dead and unable to function. For example, when you pinch yourself, you feel pain. Have you ever thought "how do I feel pain?" You might answer that it is because you have a nervous system in your body which perceives the pinch and sends a signal to the brain. However, there is more to it than that. The nervous system is material, and if it didn't have energy circulating in it, it wouldn't function. Chi is the energy which makes the nervous system and the other parts of your body work. When you pinch your skin, that area

-20-

is stimulated and the Chi field is disturbed. Your brain is designed to sense this and other disturbances, and to interpret the cause.

According to Chinese Chi Kung and medicine, the Chi in your body is divided into two categories: Managing Chi (Ying Chi)(which is often called Nutritive Chi) and Guardian Chi (Wey Chi). The Managing Chi is the energy which has been sent to the organs so that they can function. The Guardian Chi is the energy which has been sent to the surface of the body to form a shield to protect you from negative outside influences such as cold. In order to keep yourself healthy, you must learn how to manage these two Chi efficiently so they can serve you well.

Chi is classified as Yin because it can only be felt, while the physical body is classified as Yang because it can be seen. Yin is the root and source of the life which animates the Yang body (physical body) and manifests power or strength externally. Therefore, when the Chi is strong, the physical body can function properly and be healthy, and it can manifest a lot of power or strength.

In order to have a strong and healthy body, you must learn how to keep the Chi circulating in your body smoothly, and you must also learn how to build up an abundant store of Chi. In order to reach these two goals, you must first understand the Chi circulatory and storage system in your body.

Chinese doctors discovered long ago that the human body has twelve major channels and eight vessels through which the Chi circulates. The twelve channels are like rivers which distribute Chi throughout the body, and also connect the extremities (fingers and toes) to the internal organs. I would like to point out here that the "internal organs" of Chinese medicine do not necessarily correspond to the physical organs as understood in the West, but rather to a set of clinical functions similar to each other, and related to the organ system. The eight vessels, which are often referred to as the extraordinary vessels, function like reservoirs and regulate the distribution and circulation of Chi in your body.

When the Chi in the eight reservoirs is full and strong, the Chi in the rivers is strong and will be regulated efficiently. When there is stagnation in any of these twelve channels or rivers, the Chi which flows to the body's extremities and to the internal organs will be abnormal, and illness may develop. You should understand that every channel has its particular Chi flow strength, and every channel is different. All of these different levels of Chi strength are affected by your mind, the weather, the time of day, the food you have eaten, and even your mood. For example, when the weather is dry the Chi in the lungs will tend to be more positive than when it is moist. When you are angry, the Chi flow in your liver channel will be abnormal. The Chi strength in the different channels varies throughout the day in a regular cycle, and at any particular time one channel is strongest. For example, between 11 AM and 1 PM the Chi flow in the heart channel is the strongest. Furthermore, the Chi level of the same organ can be different from one person to another.

Whenever the Chi flow in the twelve rivers or channels is not normal, the eight reservoirs will regulate the Chi flow and bring it back to normal. For example, when you experience a sudden shock, the Chi flow in the bladder immediately becomes deficient. Normally the reservoir will immediately regulate the Chi in this channel so that you recover from the shock. However, if the reservoir Chi is also deficient, or if the effect of the shock is too great and there is not enough time to regulate the Chi, the bladder will suddenly contract, causing unavoidable urination.

When a person is sick because of an injury, his Chi level tends to be either too positive (excessive, Yang) or too negative (deficient, Yin). A Chinese physician would either use a prescription of herbs to adjust the Chi, or else he would insert acupuncture needles at various spots on the channels to inhibit the flow in some channels and stimulate the flow in others, so that balance can be restored. However, there is another alternative, and that is to use certain physical and mental exercises to adjust the Chi. In other words, to use Chi Kung.

In the last twenty years, Western medicine has gradually begun to accept the existence of Chi and its circulation in the human body. Several studies indicate that what the Chinese call "Chi" is the bioelectric circulation in the body. It is now generally accepted by Western medicine that imbalance of the bioelectric current is a major cause of most illness. Modern science is now learning many things which will help us to better understand Chi Kung, and will also increase Western medicine's willingness to accept the validity of Chi Kung.

If Chi is the bioelectricity circulating in the human body, in order to maintain the circulation of Chi or bioelectricity there must be an EMF (electromagnetic force) generating an electric potential difference. It is like an electric circuit, which must be hooked up to a battery or other source of EMF before there can be a current.

There are two main purposes in Chi Kung training: first, to maintain the smooth circulation of Chi (bioelectricity), and second, to fill up the Chi vessels (Chi reservoirs) with Chi. In order to have smooth circulation of Chi we must regulate the electric potential difference which controls the Chi flow, and also remove all sources of resistance in the path of the circulation. In order to fill up the Chi vessels, we need to know how to increase the charge in our "battery."

At this point you may ask, "If we keep increasing the EMF of the battery (Chi reservoirs), won't the excess Chi flow overheat the circuit (make it too Yang)?" The answer is yes, this can happen. However, your body is different from a regular electric circuit in that it is alive and can change. When the Chi flow becomes stronger, your body will react and build itself up so that it can accept this new Chi flow. Chi Kung should be trained slowly and carefully so that, as you build up the Chi stored in your channels, your body has time to readjust itself. All of this also makes your body stronger and healthier.

You can see that the key to Chi Kung practice is, in addition to removing resistance from the Chi channels, maintaining or increasing the Chi level (EMF) in the Chi reservoirs (battery). What are the energy sources in our daily life which supply energy to our body, or, expressed differently, what are the sources by which the EMF can be increased in the body's bioelectric circuit, which would increase the flow of bioelectricity? There are four major sources.

1. **Natural Energy.** Since your body is of electrically conductive material, its electromagnetic field is always affected by the sun, the moon, clouds, the earth's magnetic field, and by the other energy around you. The major influences are the sun's radiation, the moon's gravity, and the earth's magnetic field. These affect your Chi circulation significantly, and are therefore responsible for the pattern of your Chi circulation since you were formed. We are now also being greatly affected by the energy generated by modern technology, such as the electromagnetic waves generated by radios, TVs, microwave ovens, computer monitors, and many other things.

2. **Food and Air.** In order to maintain life, we take in food and air Essence through the mouth and nose. These Essences are then converted into Chi through biochemical reaction in the chest and digestive system (called Triple Burners in Chinese medicine). When the Chi is converted from the Essence, an EMF is generated which circulates the Chi throughout the body. A major part of Chi Kung is devoted to getting the proper kinds of food and fresh air.

3. **Thinking.** The human mind is the most important and efficient source of bioelectric EMF. Any time you move to do something you must first generate an idea (Yi). This idea generates the EMF and leads the Chi to energize the appropriate muscles to carry out the desired motion. The more you can concentrate, the stronger the EMF you can generate, and the stronger the flow of Chi you can lead. Naturally, the stronger the flow of Chi you lead to the muscles, the more they will be energized. Because of this, the mind is considered the most important factor in Chi Kung training.

4. **Exercise.** Exercise converts the food Essence (fat) stored in your body into Chi, and therefore builds up the EMF. Many Chi Kung styles have been created which utilize movement for this purpose.

In Tai Chi Chi Kung, the mind and the movements are the two major sources of EMF, though the other two sources are also involved. For example, when you practice in the early morning you can absorb energy from the sun. When you meditate facing the south in the evening you align yourself with the earth's magnetic field. It is also advisable to eliminate greasy and other undesirable foods from your diet, and, if possible, to practice in the mountains where the air is fresh and clear.

1-7. General Concepts of Chi Kung Training

Before you start your Chi Kung training, you must first understand the three treasures of life - Jieng (Essence), Chi (Internal Energy), and Shen (Spirit) - as well as their interrelationship. If you lack this understanding, you are missing the root of Chi Kung training, as well as the basic idea of Chi Kung theory. The main goals of Chi Kung training are to learn how to retain your Jieng, strengthen and smooth your Chi flow, and enlighten your Shen. To reach these goals you must learn how to regulate the body (Tyau Shenn), regulate the mind (Tyau Hsin), regulate the breathing (Tyau Shyi), regulate the Chi (Tyau Chi), and regulate the Shen (Tyau Shen).

Regulating the body includes understanding how to find and build the root of the body, as well as the root of the individual forms you are practicing. To build a firm root, you must know how to keep your center, how to balance your body, and most important of all, how to relax so that the Chi can flow.

Regulating the mind involves learning how to keep your mind calm, peaceful, and centered, so that you can judge situations objectively and lead Chi to the desired places. The mind is the main key to success in Chi Kung practice.

To regulate your breathing, you must learn how to breathe so that your breathing and your mind mutually correspond and cooperate. When you breathe this way, your mind will be able to attain peace more quickly, and therefore concentrate more easily on leading the Chi.

Regulating the Chi is one of the ultimate goals of Chi Kung practice. In order to regulate your Chi effectively you must first have regulated your body, mind, and breathing. Only then will your mind be clear enough to sense how the Chi is distributed in your body, and understand how to adjust it.

For Buddhist priests, who seek the enlightenment of the Buddha, regulating the Shen is the final goal of Chi Kung. This enables them to maintain a neutral, objective perspective of life, and this perspective is the eternal life of the Buddha. The average Chi Kung practitioner has lower goals. He raises his Shen in order to increase his concentration and enhance his vitality. This makes it possible for him to lead Chi effectively to his entire body so that it carries out the managing and guarding duties. This maintains his health and slows down the aging process.

If you understand these few things you will be able to quickly enter into the field of Chi Kung. Without all of these important elements, your training will be ineffective and your time will be wasted.

Three Treasures - Jieng, Chi, and Shen

Before you start any Chi Kung training you must first understand the three treasures (San Bao): Jieng (Essence), Chi (Internal Energy), and Shen (Spirit). They are also called the three origins or the three roots (San Yuan), because they are considered the origins and roots of your life. Jieng means Essence, the most original and refined part. Jieng is the original source and most basic part of every living thing, and determines its nature and characteristics. It is the root of life. Sperm is called Jieng Tzyy, which means "Essence of the Son," because it contains the Jieng of the father which is passed on to his son (or daughter) and becomes the son's Jieng.

Chi is the internal energy of your body. It is like the electricity which passes through a machine to keep it running. Chi comes either from the conversion of the Jieng which you have received from your parents, or from the food you eat and the air you breathe.

Shen is the center of your mind and being. It is what makes you human, because animals do not have a Shen. The Shen in your body must be nourished by your Chi or energy. When your Chi is full, your Shen will be enlivened.

Chinese meditators and Chi Kung practitioners believe that the body contains two general types of Chi. The first type is called Pre-birth Chi, and it comes from converted Original Jieng, which you get from your parents at conception. The second type, which is called Post-birth Chi, is drawn from the Jieng of the food and air we take in. When this Chi flows or is led to the brain, it can energize the Shen and soul. This energized and raised Shen is able to lead the Chi to the entire body.

Each one of these three elements or treasures has its own root. You must know the roots so that you can strengthen and protect your three treasures.

1. Your body requires many kinds of Jieng. Except for the Jieng which you inherent from your parents, which is called Original Jieng (Yuan Jieng), all other Jiengs must be obtained from food and air. Among all of these Jiengs, Original Jieng is the most important one. It is the root and the seed of your life, and your basic strength. If your parents were strong and healthy, your Original Jieng will be strong and healthy, and you will have a strong foundation on which to grow. The Chinese people believe that in order to stay healthy and live a long life, you must protect and maintain this Jieng.
    The root of Original Jieng (Yuan Jieng) before your birth was in your parents. After birth this Original Jieng stays in its residence - the kidneys, which are considered the root of your Jieng. When you keep this root strong, you will have sufficient Original Jieng to supply to your body. Although you cannot increase the amount of Original Jieng you have, Chi Kung training can improve the quality of your Jieng. Chi Kung can also teach you how to convert your Jieng into Original Chi more efficiently, and how to use this Chi effectively.

2. Chi is converted both from the Jieng which you have inherited from your parents and from the Jieng which you draw from the food and air you take in. Chi that is converted from the Original Jieng which you inherited is called Original Chi (Yuan

Chi).(*10) Just as Original Jieng is the most important type of Jieng, Original Chi is the most important type of Chi. It is pure and of high quality, while the Chi from food and air may make your body too positive or too negative, depending on how and where you absorb it. When you retain and protect your Original Jieng, you will be able to generate Original Chi in a pure, continuous stream. As a Chi Kung practitioner, you must know how to convert your Original Jieng into Original Chi in a smooth, steady stream.

Since your Original Chi comes from your Original Jieng, they both have the kidneys for their root. When your kidneys are strong, the Original Jieng is strong, and the Original Chi converted from this Original Jieng will also be full and strong. This Chi resides in the Lower Dan Tien in your abdomen. Once you learn how to convert your Original Jieng, you will be able to supply your body with all the Chi it needs.

3. Shen is the force which keeps you alive. It has no substance, but it gives expression and appearance to your Jieng. Shen is also the control tower for the Chi. When your Shen is strong, your Chi is strong and you can lead it efficiently. The root of Shen (Spirit) is your mind (Yi, or intention). When your brain is energized and stimulated, your mind will be more aware and you will be able to concentrate more intensely. Also, your Shen will be raised. Advanced Chi Kung practitioners believe that your brain must always be sufficiently nourished by your Chi. It is the Chi which keeps your mind clear and concentrated. With an abundant Chi supply, the mind can be energized, and can raise the Shen and enhance your vitality.

The deeper levels of Chi Kung training include the conversion of Jieng into Chi, which is then led to the brain to raise the Shen. This process is called "Faan Jieng Buu Nao" (*11) and means "return the Jieng to nourish the brain." When Chi is led to the head, it stays at the the Upper Dan Tien (center of forehead), which is the residence of your Shen. Chi and Shen are mutually related. When your Shen is weak, your Chi is weak, and your body will degenerate rapidly. Shen is the headquarters of Chi. Likewise, Chi supports the Shen, energizing it and keeping it sharp, clear, and strong. If the Chi in your body is weak, your Shen will also be weak.

(*10).Before birth you have no Chi of your own, but rather you use your mother's Chi. When you are born, you start creating Chi from the Original Jieng which you received from your parents. This Chi is called Pre-birth Chi, as well as Original Chi. It is also called Pre-heaven Chi (Shian Tian Chi) because it comes from the Original Jieng which you received before you saw the heavens (which here means the sky), i.e. before your birth.

(*11). 還精補腦

Chi Kung Training Theory

In Chi Kung training it is important to understand the principle behind everything you are doing. The principle is the root of your practice, and it is this root which brings forth the results you want. The root gives life, while the branches and flowers (results) give only temporary beauty. If you keep the root, you can regrow. If you have just branches and flowers, they will die in a short time.

Every Chi Kung form or practice has its special purpose and theory. If you do not know the purpose and theory, you have lost the root (meaning) of the practice. Therefore, as a Chi Kung practitioner, you must continue to ponder and practice until you understand the root of every set or form.

Before you start training, you must first understand that all of the training originates in your mind. You must have a clear idea of what you are doing, and your mind must be calm, centered, and balanced. This also implies that your feeling, sensing, and judgement must be objective and accurate. This requires emotional balance and a clear mind. This takes a lot of hard work, but once you have reached this level you will have built the root of your physical training, and your Yi (mind) will be able to lead your Chi throughout your physical body.

As mentioned previously, Chi Kung training includes five important elements: regulating the body, regulating the breath, regulating the Yi (Mind), regulating the Chi, and regulating the Shen (Spirit). These are the foundation of successful Chi Kung practice. Without this foundation, your understanding of Chi Kung and your practice will remain superficial.

1. Regulating the Body (Tyau Shenn) 調身

Regulating the Body is called "Tyau Shenn" in Chinese. This means to adjust your body until it is in the most comfortable and relaxed state. This implies that your body must be centered and balanced. If it is not, you will be tense and uneasy, and this will affect the judgement of your Yi and the circulation of your Chi. In Chinese medical society it is said: "(When) shape (body's posture) is not correct, then the Chi will not be smooth. (When) the Chi is not smooth, the Yi (Mind) will not be peaceful. (When) the Yi is not peaceful, then the Chi is disordered."(*12) You should understand that the relaxation of your body originates with your Yi. Therefore, before you can relax your body, you must first relax or regulate your mind (Yi). This is called "Shenn Hsin Pyng Herng,"(*13) which means "Body and heart (Mind) balanced." The body and the mind are mutually related. A relaxed and balanced body helps your Yi to relax and concentrate. When your Yi is at peace and can judge things accurately, your body will be centered, balanced, and relaxed.

(*12). 形不正，則氣不順．氣不順，則意不寧．意不寧，則氣散亂．

(*13). 身心平衡

Relaxation

Relaxation is one of the major keys to success in Chi Kung. You should remember that **ONLY WHEN YOU ARE RELAXED WILL ALL YOUR CHI CHANNELS BE OPEN**. In order to be relaxed, your Yi must first be relaxed and calm. When this Yi coordinates with your breathing, your body will be able to relax.

In Chi Kung practice there are three levels of relaxation. The first level is the external physical relaxation, or postural relaxation. This is a very superficial level, and almost anyone can reach it. It consists of adopting a comfortable stance and avoiding unnecessary strain in how you stand and move. The second level is the relaxation of the muscles and tendons. To do this your Yi must be directed deep into the muscles and tendons. This relaxation will help open your Chi channels, and will allow the Chi to sink and accumulate in the Dan Tien.

The final stage is the relaxation which reaches the internal organs and the bone marrow. Remember, **ONLY IF YOU CAN RELAX DEEP INTO YOUR BODY WILL YOUR MIND BE ABLE TO LEAD THE CHI THERE**. Only at this stage will the Chi be able to reach everywhere. Then you will feel transparent - as if your whole body had disappeared. If you can reach this level of relaxation, you will be able to communicate with your organs and use Chi Kung to adjust or regulate the Chi disorders which are giving you problems. You will also be able to protect your organs more effectively, and therefore slow down their degeneration.

Rooting

In all Chi Kung practice it is very important to be rooted. Being rooted means to be stable and in firm contact with the ground. If you want to push a car, you have to be rooted so the force you exert into the car will be balanced by a force into the ground. If you are not rooted, when you push the car you will only push yourself away, and not move the car. Your root is made up of your body's root, center, and balance.

Before you can develop your root, you must first relax and let your body "settle." As you relax, the tension in the various parts of your body will dissolve, and you will find a comfortable way to stand. You will stop fighting the ground to keep your body up, and will learn to rely on your body's structure to support itself. This lets the muscles relax even more. Since your body isn't struggling to stand up, your Yi won't be pushing upward, and your body, mind, and Chi will all be able to sink. If you let dirty water sit quietly, the impurities will gradually settle down to the bottom, leaving the water above it clear. In the same way, if you relax your body enough to let it settle, your Chi will sink to your Dan Tien and the Bubbling Wells in your feet, and your mind will become clear. Then you can begin to develop your root.

To root your body you must imitate a tree and grow an invisible root under your feet. This will give you a firm root to keep you stable in your training. **YOUR ROOT MUST BE WIDE AS WELL**

AS DEEP. Naturally, your Yi must grow first, because it is the Yi which leads the Chi. Your Yi must be able to lead the Chi to your feet, and be able to communicate with the ground. Only when your Yi can communicate with the ground will your Chi be able to grow beyond your feet and enter the ground to build the root. The Bubbling Well cavity is the gate which enables your Chi to communicate with the ground.

After you have gained your root, you must learn how to keep your center. A stable center will make your Chi develop evenly and uniformly. If you lose this center, your Chi will not be led evenly. In order to keep your body centered, you must first center your Yi, and then match your body to it. Only under these conditions will the Chi Kung forms you practice have their root. Your mental and physical center is the key which enables you to lead your Chi beyond your body.

Balance is the product of rooting and centering. Balance includes balancing the Chi and the physical body. It does not matter which aspect of balance you are dealing with, first you must balance your Yi, and only then can you balance your Chi and your physical body. If your Yi is balanced, it can help you to make accurate judgements, and therefore to correct the path of the Chi flow.

Rooting includes rooting not just the body, but also the form or movement. The root of any form or movement is found in its purpose or principle. For example, in certain Chi Kung exercises you want to lead the Chi to your palms. In order to do this you must imagine that you are pushing an object forward while keeping your muscles relaxed. In this exercise, your elbows must be down to build the sense of root for the push. If you raise the elbows, you lose the sense of "intention" of the movement, because the push would be ineffective if you were pushing something for real. Since the intention or purpose of the movement is its reason for being, you now have a purposeless movement, and you have no reason to lead Chi in any particular way. Therefore, in this case, the elbow is the root of the movement.

2. Regulating the Breath (Tyau Shyi) 調息

Regulating the breath means to regulate your breathing until it is calm, smooth, and peaceful. Only when you have reached this point will you be able to make the breathing deep, slender, long, and soft, which is required for successful Chi Kung practice.

Breathing is affected by your emotions. For example, when you are angry you exhale more strongly than you inhale. When you are sad, you inhale more strongly than you exhale. When your mind is peaceful and calm, your inhalation and exhalation are relatively equal. In order to keep your breathing calm, peaceful, and steady, your mind and emotions must first be calm and neutral. Therefore, in order to regulate your breathing, you must first regulate your mind.

The other side of the coin is that you can use your breathing to control your Yi. When your breathing is uniform, it is as if you were hypnotizing your Yi, which helps to calm it. You can see that Yi and breathing are interdependent, and that they cooperate with each other. Deep and calm breathing relaxes you and keeps your mind clear. It fills your lungs with plenty of air, so that your brain and entire body have an adequate supply of oxygen. In addition, deep and complete breathing enables the diaphragm to move up and down, which massages and stimulates the internal organs. For this reason, deep breathing exercises are also called "internal organ exercises."

Deep and complete breathing does not mean that you inhale and exhale to the maximum. This would cause the lungs and the surrounding muscles to tense up, which in turn would keep the air from circulating freely, and hinder the absorption of oxygen. Without enough oxygen, your mind becomes scattered, and the rest of your body tenses up. In correct breathing, you inhale and exhale to about 70% or 80% of capacity, so that your lungs stay relaxed.

You can conduct an easy experiment. Inhale deeply so that your lungs are completely full, and time how long you can hold your breath. Then try inhaling to only about 70% of your capacity, and see how long you can hold your breath. You will find that with the latter method you can last much longer than with the first one. This is simply because the lungs and the surrounding muscles are relaxed. When they are relaxed, the rest of your body and your mind can also relax, which significantly decreases your need for oxygen. Therefore, when you regulate your breathing, the first priority is to keep your lungs relaxed and calm.

When training, your mind must first be calm so that your breathing can be regulated. When the breathing is regulated, your mind is able to reach a higher level of calmness. This calmness can again help you to regulate the breathing, until your mind is deep. After you have trained for a long time, your breathing will be full and slender, and your mind will be very clear. It is said: "Hsin Shyi Shiang Yi,"(*14) which means "Heart (Mind) and breathing (are) mutually dependent." When you reach this meditative state, your heartbeat slows down, and your mind is very clear: you have entered the sphere of real meditation.

An Ancient Taoist named Li Ching-Yen said: "Regulating breathing means to regulate the real breathing until (you) stop."(*15) This means that correct regulating means not regulating. In other words, although you start by consciously regulating your breath, you must get to the point where the regulating happens naturally, and you no longer have to think about it. When you breathe, if you concentrate your mind on your breathing, then it is not true regulating, because the Chi in your lungs will become stagnant. When you reach the level of true regulating, you don't have to pay attention to it, and you can use your mind efficiently to lead the Chi. Remember **WHEREVER THE YI IS, THERE IS THE CHI. IF THE YI STOPS IN ONE SPOT, THE CHI WILL BE STAGNANT.**

(*14). 心息相依
(*15). 調息要調無息息

IT IS THE YI WHICH LEADS THE CHI AND MAKES IT MOVE.
Therefore, when you are in a state of correct breath regulation, your mind is free. There is no sound, stagnation, urgency, or hesitation, and you can finally be calm and peaceful.

You can see that when the breath is regulated correctly, the Chi will also be regulated. They are mutually related and cannot be separated. This idea is explained frequently in Taoist literature. The Taoist Goang Cherng Tzyy said: "One exhale, the Earth Chi rises; one inhale, the Heaven Chi descends; real man's (meaning one who has attained the real Tao) repeated breathing at the navel, then my real Chi is naturally connected."(*16) This says that when you breathe you should move your abdomen, as if you were breathing from your navel. The earth Chi is the negative (Yin) energy from your kidneys, and the sky Chi is the positive (Yang) energy which comes from the food you eat and the air you breathe. When you breathe from the navel, these two Chi's will connect and combine. Some people think that they know what Chi is, but they really don't. Once you connect the two Chi's, you will know what the "real" Chi is, and you may become a "real" man, which means to attain the Tao.

The Taoist book Chain Tao Jen Yen (Sing (of the) Tao (with) Real Words) says: "One exhale one inhale to communicate Chi's function, one movement one calmness is the same as (i.e., is the source of) creation and variation."(*17) The first part of this statement again implies that the functioning of Chi is connected with the breathing. The second part of this sentence means that all creation and variation come from the interaction of movement (Yang) and calmness (Yin). Hwang Tyng Ching (Yellow Yard Classic) says: "Breathe Original Chi to seek immortality."(*18) In China, the traditional Taoists wore yellow robes, and they meditated in a "yard" or hall. This sentence means that in order to reach the goal of immortality, you must seek to find and understand the Original Chi which comes from the Dan Tien through correct breathing.

Moreover, the Taoist Wuu Jen Ren said: "Use the Post-birth breathing to look for the real person's (i.e. the immortal's) breathing place."(*19) In this sentence it is clear that in order to locate the immortal breathing place (the Dan Tien), you must rely on and know how to regulate your Post-birth, or natural, breathing. Through regulating your Post-birth breathing you will gradually be able to locate the residence of the Chi (the Dan Tien), and eventually you will be able to use your Dan Tien to breath like the immortal

---

(*16). 廣成子曰：" 一呼則地氣上升，一吸則天氣下
降，人之反覆呼吸於蒂，則我之真氣自然相接
。"

(*17). 唱道真言曰：" 一呼一吸通乎氣機，一動一靜
同乎造化．"

(*18). 黃庭經曰：" 呼吸元氣以求仙．"

(*19). 靈源大道歌曰：" 元和內運即成真，呼吸外求
終未了．"

Taoists. Finally, in the Taoist song Ling Yuan Dah Tao Ge (The Great Taoist Song of the Spirit's Origin) it is said: "The Originals (Original Jieng, Chi, and Shen) are internally transported peacefully, so that you can become real (immortal); (if you) depend (only) on external breathing (you) will not reach the end (goal)."(*20) From this song, you can see that internal breathing (breathing at the Dan Tien) is the key to training your three treasures and finally reaching immortality. However, you must first know how to regulate your external breathing correctly.

All of these emphasize the importance of breathing. There are eight key words for air breathing which a Chi Kung practitioner should follow during his practice. Once you understand them you will be able to substantially shorten the time needed to reach your Chi Kung goals. These eight key words are: 1. Calm (Jing); 2. Slender (Shyi); 3. Deep (Shenn); 4. Long (Charng); 5. Continuous (Iou): 6. Uniform (Yun); 7. Slow (Hoan), and 8. Soft (Mian). These key words are self-explanatory, and with a little thought you should be able to understand them.

3. Regulating the Mind (Tyau Hsin) 調心

It is said in Taoist society that: "(When) large Tao is taught, first stop thought; when thought is not stopped, (the lessons are) in vain."(*21) This means that when you first practice Chi Kung, the most difficult training is to stop your thinking. The final goal for your mind is "the thought of no thought."(*22) Your mind does not think of the past, the present, or the future. Your mind is completely separated from influences of the present such as worry, happiness, and sadness. Then your mind can be calm and steady, and can finally gain peace. Only when you are in the state of "the thought of no thought" will you be relaxed and able to sense calmly and accurately.

Regulating your mind means using your consciousness to stop the activity in your mind in order to set it free from the bondage of ideas, emotion, and conscious thought. When you reach this level your mind will be calm, peaceful, empty, and light. Then your mind has really reached the goal of relaxation. Only when you reach this stage will you be able to relax deep into your marrow and internal organs. Only then will your mind be clear enough to see (feel) the internal Chi circulation and to communicate with your Chi and organs. In Taoist society it is called "Nei Shyh Kung Fu,"(*23) which means the Kung Fu of internal vision.

When you reach this real relaxation you may be able to sense the different elements which make up your body: solid matter, liquids, gases, energy, and spirit. You may even be able to see or feel the dif-

---

(*20). 靈源大道歌曰： ＂元和內運即成真，呼吸外求
終末了．＂
(*21). 大道教人先止念，念頭不住亦徒然．
(*22). 無念之念
(*23). 內視功夫

-32-

ferent colors that are associated with your five organs - green (liver), white (lungs), black (kidneys), yellow (spleen), and red (heart).

Once your mind is relaxed and regulated and you can sense your internal organs, you may decide to study the five element theory. This is a very profound subject, and it is sometimes interpreted differently by Oriental physicians and Chi Kung practitioners. When understood properly, it can give you a method of analyzing the interrelationships between your organs, and help you devise ways to correct imbalances.

For example, the lungs correspond to the element Metal, and the heart to the element Fire. Metal (the lungs) can be used to adjust the heat of the Fire (the heart), because metal can take a large quantity of heat away from fire, (and thus cool down the heart). When you feel uneasy or have heartburn (excess fire in the heart), you may use deep breathing to calm down the uneasy emotions or cool off the heartburn.

Naturally, it will take a lot of practice to reach this level. In the beginning, you should not have any ideas or intentions, because they will make it harder for your mind to relax and empty itself of thoughts. Once you are in a state of "no thought," place your attention on your Dan Tien. It is said "Yi Shoou Dan Tien,"(*24) which means "The Mind is kept on the Dan Tien." The Dan Tien is the origin and residence of your Chi. Your mind can build up the Chi here (start the fire, Chii Huoo), then lead the Chi anywhere you wish, and finally lead the Chi back to its residence. When your mind is on the Dan Tien, your Chi will always have a root. When you keep this root, your Chi will be strong and full, and it will go where you want it to. You can see that when you practice Chi Kung, your mind cannot be completely empty and relaxed. You must find the firmness within the relaxation, then you can reach your goal.

In Chi Kung training, it is said: "Use your Yi (Mind) to **LEAD** your Chi" (Yii Yi Yiin Chi)(*25). Notice the word **LEAD**. Chi behaves like water - it cannot be pushed, but it can be led. When Chi is led, it will flow smoothly and without stagnation. When it is pushed, it will flood and enter the wrong paths. Remember, wherever your Yi goes first, the Chi will naturally follow. For example, if you intend to lift an object, this intention is your Yi. This Yi will lead the Chi to the arms to energize the physical muscles, and then the object can be lifted.

It is said: "Your Yi cannot be on your Chi. Once your Yi is on your Chi, the Chi is stagnant."(*26) When you want to walk from one spot to another, you must first mobilize your intention and direct it to the goal, then your body will follow. The mind must always be ahead of the body. If your mind stays on your body, you will not be able to move.

(*24). 意守丹田

(*25). 以意引氣

(*26). 意不在氣，在氣則滯.

In Chi Kung training, the first thing is to know what Chi is. If you do not know what Chi is, how will you be able to lead it? Once you know what Chi is and experience it, then your Yi will have something to lead. The next thing in Chi Kung training is knowing how your Yi communicates with your Chi. That means that your Yi should be able to sense and feel the Chi flow and understand how strong and smooth it is. In Tai Chi Chi Kung society, it is commonly said that your Yi must "listen" to your Chi and "understand" it. Listen means to pay careful attention to what you sense and feel. The more you pay attention, the better you will be able to understand. Only after you understand the Chi situation will your Yi be able to set up the strategy. In Chi Kung your mind or Yi must generate the idea (visualize your intention), which is like an order to your Chi to complete a certain mission.

The more your Yi communicates with your Chi, the more efficiently the Chi can be led. For this reason, as a Chi Kung beginner you must first learn about Yi and Chi, and also learn how to help them communicate efficiently. Yi is the key in Chi Kung practice. Without this Yi you would not be able to lead your Chi, let alone build up the strength of the Chi or circulate it throughout your entire body.

Remember **WHEN THE YI IS STRONG, THE CHI IS STRONG, AND WHEN THE YI IS WEAK, THE CHI IS WEAK**. Therefore, the first step of Chi Kung training is to develop your Yi. The first secret of a strong Yi is **CALMNESS**. When you are calm, you can see things clearly and not be disturbed by surrounding distractions. With your mind calm, you will be able to concentrate.

Confucius said: "First you must be calm, then your mind can be steady. Once your mind is steady, then you are at peace. Only when you are at peace are you able to think and finally gain."(*27) This procedure is also applied in meditation or Chi Kung exercise: First Calm, then Steady, Peace, Think, and finally Gain. When you practice Chi Kung, first you must learn to be emotionally calm. Once calm, you will be able to see what you want and firm your mind (steady). This firm and steady mind is your intention or Yi (it is how your Yi is generated). Only after you know what you really want will your mind gain peace and be able to relax emotionally and physically. Once you have reached this step, you must then concentrate or think in order to execute your intention. Under this thoughtful and concentrated mind, your Chi will follow and you will be able to gain what you wish.

4. Regulating the Chi (Tyau Chi) 調氣

Before you can regulate your Chi you must first regulate your body, breath, and mind. If you compare your body to a battlefield, then your mind is like the general who generates ideas and controls the situation, and your breathing is the strategy. Your Chi is like the soldiers who are led to the most advantageous places on the battlefield. All

(*27). 孔子曰： ＂先靜爾後有定，定爾後能安，安爾
後能慮，慮爾後能得．＂

-34-

four elements are necessary, and all four must be coordinated with each other if you are to win the war against sickness and aging.

If you want to arrange your soldiers most effectively for battle, you must know which area of the battlefield is most important, and where you are weakest (where your Chi is deficient) and need to send reinforcements. If you have more soldiers than you need in one area (excessive Chi), then you can send them somewhere else where the ranks are thin. As a general, you must also know how many soldiers are available for the battle, and how many you will need for protecting yourself and your headquarters. To be successful, not only do you need good strategy (breathing), but you also need to communicate and understand the situation effectively with your troops, or all of your strategy will be in vain. When your Yi (the general) knows how to regulate the body (knows the battlefield), how to regulate the breathing (set up the strategy), and how to effectively regulate the Chi (direct your soldiers), you will be able to reach the final goal of Chi Kung training.

In order to regulate your Chi so that it moves smoothly in the correct paths, you need more than just efficient Yi-Chi communication. You also need to know how to generate Chi. If you do not have enough Chi in your body, how can you regulate it? In a battle, if you do not have enough soldiers to set up your strategy, you have already lost.

When you practice Chi Kung, you must first train to make your Chi flow naturally and smoothly. There are some Chi Kung exercises in which you intentionally hold your Yi, and thus hold your Chi, in a specific area. As a beginner, however, you should first learn how to make the Chi flow smoothly instead of building a Chi dam, which is commonly done in external martial Chi Kung training.

In order to make Chi flow naturally and smoothly, your Yi must first be relaxed. Only when your Yi is relaxed will your body be relaxed and the Chi channels open for the Chi to circulate. Then you must coordinate your Chi flow with your breathing. Breathing regularly and calmly will make your Yi calm, and allow your body to relax even more.

5. Regulating Spirit (Tyau Shen) 調神

There is one thing that is more important than anything else in a battle, and that is fighting spirit. You may have the best general, who knows the battlefield well and is also an expert strategist, but if his soldiers do not have a high fighting spirit (morale), he might still lose. Remember, **SPIRIT IS THE CENTER AND ROOT OF A FIGHT**. When you keep this center, one soldier can be equal to ten soldiers. When his spirit is high, a soldier will obey his orders accurately and willingly, and his general will be able to control the situation efficiently. In a battle, in order for a soldier to have this kind of morale, he must know why he is fighting, how to fight, and what he can expect after the fight. Under these conditions, he will know what he is doing and why, and this understanding will raise up his spirit, strengthen his will, and increase his patience and endurance.

It is the same with Chi Kung training. In order to reach the final goal of Chi Kung you must have three fundamental spiritual roots: will, patience, and endurance.

Shen, which is the Chinese term for spirit, originates from the Yi (the general). When the Shen is strong, the Yi is firm. When the Yi is firm, the Shen will be steady and calm. **THE SHEN IS THE MENTAL PART OF A SOLDIER. WHEN THE SHEN IS HIGH, THE CHI IS STRONG AND EASILY DIRECTED. WHEN THE CHI IS STRONG, THE SHEN IS ALSO STRONG.**

All of these training concepts and procedures are common to all Chinese Chi Kung, and you should also adhere to them when practicing Tai Chi Chuan. To reach a deep level of understanding and penetrate to the essence of any Chi Kung practice, you should always keep these five training criteria in mind and examine them for deeper levels of meaning. This is the only way to gain the real mental and physical health benefits from your training. Always remember that Chi Kung training is not just the forms. Your feelings and comprehension are the essential roots of the entire training. This Yin side of the training has no limit, and the deeper you understand, the more you will see that there is to know.

1-8. Tai Chi Chuan and Chi Kung
The previous discussion can be summarized as follows:

1. Tai Chi was originally created as a martial arts style, and was used in combat. Chi Kung training was necessary for reaching the highest levels of fighting ability.

2. Tai Chi Chi Kung is only one style of martial Chi Kung, and martial Chi Kung is only one category of Chinese Chi Kung. Many of the Tai Chi Chi Kung movements were adapted from Tai Chi Chuan forms.

3. Tai Chi Chi Kung is different from many other martial Chi Kung systems in that it emphasizes the soft and builds up Chi internally through Nei Dan practice, although it also practices Wai Dan through the soft body movements. This is different from many other martial Chi Kung styles which are relatively harder physically and emphasize Wai Dan practice.

4. In the last fifty years, Tai Chi Chi Kung has been practiced mainly for health purposes, rather than martial ones.

Next, in order to understand Tai Chi Chi Kung, we should analyze the reasons for training.

1. To help Tai Chi beginners feel their Chi. Beginners usually do not have even the slightest concept of Chi. Tai Chi Chi Kung gradually gives them an understanding of Chi through feeling and experiencing it. This kind of knowledge is necessary for any kind of advancement in Tai Chi. For this reason, Tai Chi beginners are usually taught some of the many simple Wai Dan forms.

2. To teach Tai Chi beginners how to regulate the body, breathing, and Yi. Once you have grasped the idea of Chi, you then start to learn how to regulate your body. This includes how to relax the body from the skin to as deep as the internal organs and bone marrow. Through this relaxation you are able to feel and sense your center, balance, and root. You must also learn how to regulate your breathing - normal abdominal breathing for relaxation and reverse abdominal breathing for Chi expansion and condensation. Most important of all, you must learn how to regulate your mind until it can be calm and concentrated without disturbance. All of these criteria are the critical keys to the correct practice of Tai Chi Chuan. If you start learning the Tai Chi sequence without having already done this basic training, you will be preoccupied with the complicated movements, and will only be able to perform them in a superficial way.

3. To teach Tai Chi beginners how to use their Yi to lead the Chi efficiently. Once you have regulated your body, breathing, and mind, you will then be able to use your concentrated mind to lead the Chi to circulate smoothly and effectively.

4. To teach Tai Chi practitioners how to circulate Chi in the 12 primary Chi channels and fill up the two main Chi vessels. If you are able to use your mind to lead the Chi efficiently, you have completed the basic Tai Chi training. This is then the time for Tai Chi forms or sequence training. In addition, you should continue your Tai Chi Chi Kung training and learn how to build up your concentration to a higher level, and consequently build your Chi to a higher level. In addition, you should also learn how to increase the Chi in the two main vessels - the Yin Conception Vessel and the Yang Governing Vessel. Still meditation is normally used for this.

5. To teach Tai Chi practitioners how to expand their Chi to the surface of the skin and to condense the Chi to the bone marrow. When the body's Chi has been built to a higher level you then start learning how to lead the Chi to the skin to increase the skin's sensitivity and into the bones to nourish the marrow.

6. To teach Tai Chi practitioners how to use the Chi to energize the muscles for maximum Jing manifestation. When you are able to lead the Chi to the skin and condense it to the marrow efficiently, you can then use this Chi to energize the muscles to a high level. This is the secret to internal Jing (Nei Jing). Internal Jing is the foundation and root of external Jing (Wai Jing).

7. To lead the advanced Tai Chi practitioner into the domain of spiritual cultivation. The ultimate goal of Tai Chi Chi Kung practice is to lead you into the domain of emptiness where your whole being is in the Wu Chi (no extremity) state. When you have reached this goal, the Chi in your body and the Chi in

nature will unite and become one, and all human desires will gradually disappear.

Although many Tai Chi masters have created Chi Kung forms, most of the training forms used today have been adopted from the Tai Chi sequence. For example, push, crane spreads its wings, wave hands in clouds, etc. are commonly used for Chi Kung training.

In order to understand why Tai Chi Chuan has become more popular than any other style of Chi Kung, you must first understand the differences between Tai Chi Chi Kung and most other Chi Kung systems:

1. Because Tai Chi Chuan was originally created for martial purposes, every movement has its defensive or offensive purpose. This means that the intention of the Yi must be strong in every movement. This enables the practitioner to lead the Chi more strongly and efficiently to the limbs, internal organs, and marrow. Because of this heavy emphasis on Yi, the Chi flow can be more fluid, and the Chi can be increased more than with the usual Chi Kung practices that do not emphasize the Yi as strongly.

2. In order to manifest Tai Chi Jing power effectively and efficiently, the Jing must first be stored. Storing Jing (in the Yi, Chi, and posture) is Yin, while manifesting Jing is Yang. Tai Chi emphasizes the Yin side and the Yang side equally, and can consequently balance Yin and Yang in the body and avoid unhealthy extremes. This is different from many other Chi Kung practices which emphasize the Yang side more than the Yin side. Practitioners who emphasize the Yang training will not get sick easily, but, because their bodies become Yang, they will age more quickly than normal.

3. Tai Chi Chi Kung includes both Nei Dan and Wai Dan training, and is more complete than those Chi Kung systems which emphasize only one or the other.

4. Tai Chi Chi Kung builds not only the Chi circulation in the primary Chi channels, but also the Guardian Chi in the skin and the marrow Chi in the bones. In addition, Tai Chi Chi Kung also teaches the practitioner how to increase the level of Chi storage and circulation in the two major vessels - the Conception and Governing Vessels.

5. Tai Chi is soft, and does not use the muscular tension which most other martial Chi Kung styles use to some degree. Tai Chi Chi Kung emphasizes using the Yi to lead Chi in a relaxed body, and does not use tension to energize the muscles. This makes it easier for the practitioner to reach a calm, peaceful, meditative state. The practitioner is able to release mental stress and physical tension, and reach a higher level of relaxation. This is the key to maintaining and improving mental and physical health.

1-9. How to Use This Book

When you practice any Chi Kung, you must first ask: What, Why, and How. "What" means: "What am I looking for?" "What do I expect?" and "What should I do?" Then you must ask: "Why do I need it?" "Why does it work?" "Why must I do it this way instead of that way?." Finally, you must determine: "How does it work?" "How much have I advanced toward my goal?" And "How will I be able to advance further?"

It is very important to understand what you are practicing, and not just automatically repeat all that you have learned. Understanding is the root of any work. With understanding you will be able to know your goal. Once you know your goal, your mind can be firm and steady. With this understanding, you will be able to see why something has happened, and what the principles and theories behind it are. Without all of this, your work will be done blindly, and it will be a long and painful process. Only when you are sure what your target is and why you need to reach it should you raise the question of how you are going to do it. The answers to all of these questions form the root of your practice, and will help you to avoid the wondering and confusion that uncertainty brings. If you keep this root, you will be able to apply the theory and make it grow - you will know how to create. Without this root, what you learn will be only branches and flowers, and in time they will wither.

In China there is a story about an old man who was able to change a piece of rock into gold. One day, a boy came to see him and asked for his help. The old man said: "Boy! What do you want? Gold? I can give you all of the gold you want." The boy replied: "No, Master, what I want is not your gold, what I want is the trick of how to change the rock into gold!" When you just have gold, you can spend it all and become poor again. If you have the trick of how to make gold, you will never be poor. For the same reason, when you learn Chi Kung you should learn the theory and principle behind it, not just the practice. Understanding theory and principle will not only shorten your time of pondering and practice, but also enable you to practice most efficiently.

One of the hardest parts of the training process is learning how to actually do the forms correctly. Every Chi Kung movement has its special meaning and purpose. In order to make sure your movements or forms are correct, it is best to work with the tape and book together. There are some important things which you may not be able to pick up from reading, but once you see them, they will be clear. An example is the transition movements between the forms. Naturally, there are other important ideas which are impossible to take the time to explain in the videotape, such as the theory and principles; these can only be explained in a book. It cannot be denied that under the tutelage of a master you can learn more quickly and perfectly than is possible using only tapes and books. What you are missing is the master's experience and feeling. However, if you ponder carefully and practice patiently and perseveringly, you will be able to make up for this lack through your own experience and practice. This book and tape are designed for self-instruction. You will find that they will serve you as a key to enter into the field of Chi Kung.

To conclude, you must practice with perseverance and patience. You need a strong will and a great deal of self-discipline. As mentioned earlier, you may find many different versions of Tai Chi Chi Kung taught by different masters. Do not be confused by all of these versions. You should understand that it does not matter which version you practice, the basic theory and principles remain the same. The most important thing is to build up the depth of your theoretical understanding so that your mind will be clear and you will understand where you are going.

Chapter 2
The Root of Tai Chi Chuan
Yin and Yang

The theory of Yin and Yang is the root of Tai Chi Chuan, and the source from which it was created and formalized. The Chi Kung sets, which are an essential part of the practice of Tai Chi, are also based on this theory. It is therefore desirable to understand Yin-Yang theory so that you can have a clear concept of what you are trying to accomplish in your practice.

2-1. The Concept of Yin and Yang, Kan and Lii

Yin and Yang

The Chinese have long believed that the universe is made up of two opposite forces - Yin and Yang - which must balance each other. When these two forces begin to lose their balance, nature finds a way to rebalance them. If the imbalance is significant, disaster will occur. However, when these two forces combine and interact with each other smoothly and harmoniously, they manifest power and generate the millions of living things.

Yin and Yang theory is also applied to the three great natural powers: heaven, earth, and man. For example, if the Yin and Yang forces of heaven (i.e., energy which comes to us from the sky) are losing balance, there can be tornados, hurricanes, or other natural disasters. When the Yin and Yang forces loose their balance on earth, rivers can change their paths and earthquakes can occur. When the Yin and Yang forces in the human body lose their balance, sickness and even death can occur. Experience has shown that the Yin and Yang balance in man is affected by the Yin and Yang balances of the earth and heaven. Similarly, the Yin and Yang balance of the earth is influenced by the heaven's Yin and Yang. Therefore, if you wish to have a healthy body and live a long life, you need to know how to adjust your body's Yin and Yang, and how to coordinate your Chi with the Yin and Yang energy of heaven and earth. The study of Yin and Yang in the human body is the root of Chinese medicine and Chi Kung.

The Chinese have classified everything in the universe according to Yin and Yang. Even feelings, thoughts, strategy, and the spirit are covered. For example, female is Yin and male is Yang, night is Yin and day is Yang, weak is Yin and strong is Yang, backward is Yin and forward is Yang, sad is Yin and happy is Yang, defense is Yin and offense is Yang, and so on.

Practitioners of Chinese medicine and Chi Kung believe that they must seek to understand the Yin and Yang of nature and the human body before they can adjust and regulate the body's energy balance into a more harmonious state. Only then can health be maintained and the causes of sickness be corrected.

Now let us discuss how Yin and Yang are defined, and how the concept of Yin and Yang is applied to the Chi circulating in the human body. Many people, even some Chi Kung practitioners, are still confused by this. When it is said that Chi can be either Yin or Yang, it does not mean that there are two different kinds of Chi like male and female, fire and water, or positive and negative charges. Chi is energy, and energy itself does not have Yin and Yang. It is like the energy which is generated from the sparking of negative and positive charges. Charges have the potential of generating energy, but are not the energy itself.

When it is said that Chi is Yin or Yang, it means that the Chi is too strong or too weak for a particular circumstance. It is relative and not absolute. Naturally, this implies that the potential which generates the Chi is strong or weak. For example, the Chi from the sun is Yang Chi, and Chi from the moon is Yin Chi. This is because the sun's energy is Yang in comparison to Human Chi, while the moon's is Yin. In any discussion of energy where people are involved, Human Chi is used as the standard. People are always especially interested in what concerns them directly, so it is natural that we are interested primarily in Human Chi and tend to view all Chi from the perspective of human Chi. This is not unlike looking at the universe from the perspective of the Earth.

When we look at the Yin and Yang of Chi within and in regard to the human body, however, we must redefine our point of reference. For example, when a person is dead, his residual Human Chi (Goe Chi or ghost Chi) is weak compared to a living person's. Therefore, the ghost's Chi is Yin while the living person's is Yang. When discussing Chi within the body, in the Lung channel for example, the reference point is the normal, healthy status of the Chi there. If the Chi is stronger than it is in the normal state, it is Yang, and, naturally, if it is weaker than this, it is Yin. There are twelve parts of the human body that are considered organs in Chinese medicine, six of them are Yin and six are Yang. The Yin organs are the Heart, Lungs, Kidneys, Liver, Spleen, and Pericardium, and the Yang organs are Large

Intestine, Small Intestine, Stomach, Gall Bladder, Urinary Bladder, and Triple Burner. Generally speaking, the Chi level of the Yin organs is lower than that of the Yang organs. The Yin organs store Original Essence and process the Essence obtained from food and air, while the Yang organs handle digestion and excretion.

When the Chi in any of your organs is not in its normal state, you feel uncomfortable. If it is very much off from the normal state, the organ will start to malfunction and you may become sick. When this happens, the Chi in your entire body will also be affected and you will feel too Yang, perhaps feverish, or too Yin, such as the weakness after diarrhea.

Your body's Chi level is also affected by natural circumstances such as the weather, climate, and seasonal changes. Therefore, when the body's Chi level is classified, the reference point is the level which feels most comfortable for those particular circumstances. Naturally, each of us is a little bit different, and what feels best and most natural for one person may be a bit different from what is right for another person. That is why the doctor will usually ask "how do you feel?" It is according to your own standard that you are judged.

Breath is closely related to the state of your Chi, and therefore also considered Yin or Yang. When you exhale you expel air from your lungs, your mind moves outward, and the Chi around the body expands. In the Chinese martial arts, the exhale is generally used to expand the Chi to energize the muscles during an attack. Therefore, you can see that the exhale is Yang - it is expanding, offensive, and strong. Naturally, based on the same theory, the inhale is considered Yin.

Your breathing is closely related to your emotions. When you lose your temper, your breathing is short and fast, i.e. Yang. When you are sad, your body is more Yin, and you inhale more than you exhale in order to absorb the Chi from the air to balance the body's Yin and bring the body back into balance. When you are excited and happy your body is Yang, and your exhale is longer than your inhale to get rid of the excess Yang which is caused by the excitement.

As mentioned before, your mind is also closely related to your Chi. Therefore, when your Chi is Yang, your mind is usually also Yang (excited) and vice versa. The mind can also be classified according to the Chi which generated it. The mind (Yi) which is generated from the calm and peaceful Chi obtained from Original Essence is considered Yin. The mind (Hsin) which originates with the food and air Essence is emotional, scattered, and excited, and it is considered Yang. The spirit, which is related to the Chi, can also be classified as Yang or Yin based on its origin.

Do not confuse Yin Chi and Yang Chi with Fire Chi and Water Chi. When the Yin and Yang of Chi are mentioned, it refers to the level of Chi according to some reference point. However, when Water and Fire Chi are mentioned, it refers to the quality of the Chi. If you are interested in reading more about the Yin and Yang of Chi, please refer to Dr. Yang's "The Root of Chinese Chi Kung" and "Muscle/-Tendon Changing and Marrow/Brain Washing Chi Kung."

Kan and Lii

The terms Kan and Lii occur frequently in Chi Kung documents. In the Eight Trigrams Kan represents "Water" while Lii represents "Fire." However, the everyday terms for water and fire are also often used. Kan and Lii training has long been of major importance to Chi Kung practitioners. In order to understand why, you must understand these two words, and the theory behind them.

First you should understand that though Kan-Lii and Yin-Yang are related, Kan and Lii are not Yin and Yang. Kan is Water, which is able to cool your body down and make it more Yin, while Lii is Fire, which warms your body and makes it more Yang. Kan and Lii are the methods or causes, while Yin and Yang are the results. When Kan and Lii are adjusted or regulated correctly, Yin and Yang will be balanced and interact harmoniously.

Chi Kung practitioners believe that your body is always too Yang, unless you are sick or have not eaten for a long time, in which case your body may be more Yin. Since your body is always Yang, it is degenerating and burning out. It is believed that this is the cause of aging. If you are able to use Water to cool down your body, you will be able to slow down the degeneration process and thereby lengthen your life. This is the main reason why Chinese Chi Kung practitioners have been studying ways of improving the quality of the Water in their bodies, and of reducing the quantity of the Fire. I believe that as a Chi Kung practitioner you should always keep this subject at the top of your list for study and research. If you earnestly ponder and experiment, you will be able to grasp the trick of adjusting them.

If you want to learn how to adjust them, you must understand that Water and Fire mean many things in your body. The first concerns your Chi. Chi is classified as Fire or Water. When your Chi is not pure and causes your physical body to heat up and your mental/spiritual body to become unstable (Yang), it is classified as Fire Chi. The Chi which is pure and is able to cool both your physical and spiritual bodies (make them more Yin) is considered Water Chi. However, your body can never be purely Water. Water can cool down the Fire, but it must never totally quench it, because then you would be dead. It is also said that Fire Chi is able to agitate and stimulate the emotions, and from these emotions generate a "mind." This mind is called Hsin, and is considered the Fire mind, Yang mind, or emotional mind. On the other hand, the mind that Water Chi generates is calm, steady, and wise. This mind is called Yi, and is considered to be the Water mind or wisdom mind. If your spirit is nourished by Fire Chi, although your spirit may be high, it will be scattered and confused (a Yang spirit). Naturally, if the spirit is nourished and raised up by Water Chi, it will be firm and steady (a Yin mind). When your Yi is able to govern your emotional Hsin effectively, your will (strong emotional intention) can be firm.

You can see from this discussion that your Chi is the main cause of the Yin and Yang of your physical body, your mind, and your spirit. To regulate your body's Yin and Yang, you must learn how to regulate your body's Water and Fire Chi, but in order to do this efficiently you must know their sources.

Once you have grasped the concepts of Yin-Yang and Kan-Lii, then you have to think about how to adjust Kan and Lii so that you can balance the Yin and Yang in your body.

Theoretically, a Chi Kung practitioner would like to keep his body in a state of Yin-Yang balance, which means the "center" point of the Yin and Yang forces. This center point is commonly called "Wu Chi" (no extremities). It is believed that Wu Chi is the original, natural state where Yin and Yang are not distinguished. In the Wu Chi state, nature is peaceful and calm. In the Wu Chi state, all of the Yin and Yang forces have gradually combined harmoniously and disappeared. When this Wu Chi theory is applied to human beings, it is the final goal of Chi Kung practice where your mind is neutral and absolutely calm. The Wu Chi state makes it possible for you to find the origin of your life, and to combine your Chi with the Chi of nature.

The ultimate goal and purpose of Tai Chi Chi Kung and Tai Chi Chuan is to find this peaceful and natural state. In order to reach this goal, you must first understand your body's Yin and Yang so that you can balance them by adjusting your Kan and Lii. Only when your Yin and Yang are balanced will you be able to find the center balance point, the Wu Chi state.

Theoretically, between the two extremes of Yin and Yang are millions of paths (i.e., different Kan and Lii methods) which can lead you to the neutral center. This accounts for the hundreds of different styles of Chi Kung which have been created over the years. You can see that the theory of Yin and Yang and the methods of Kan and Lii are the root of training in all Chinese Chi Kung styles. Without this root, the essence of Chi Kung practice would be lost.

2-2. Yin and Yang in Tai Chi Chuan

In Wang Tzong-Yeuh's Tai Chi Classic he states "What is Tai Chi? It is generated from Wu Chi. It is the mother of Yin and Yang. When it moves, it divides. At rest it reunites"(*1). According to Chinese Taoist scripture, the universe was initially without life. The world had just cooled down from its fiery creation and all was foggy and blurry, without differentiation or separation, with no extremities or ends. This state was called "Wu Chi" (literally "no extremity"). Later, the existing natural energy divided into two extremes, known as Yin and Yang. This polarity is called Tai Chi, which means "Grand Ultimate" or "Grand Extremity," and also means "Very Ultimate" or "Very Extreme." It is this initial separation which allows and causes all other separations and changes.

You can see from this explanation that Tai Chi (Grand Ultimate) is not Wu Chi. Tai Chi is produced from Wu Chi and is

(*1). 王宗岳：" 太极者，無极而生，陰陽之母也，
動之則分，靜之則合 ．"

-45-

the mother of Yin and Yang. This means that Tai Chi is the process which is between Wu Chi and Yin and Yang. Then what is Tai Chi? It is the hidden force which is able to lead Wu Chi into the division of Yin and Yang, and also to lead the divided Yin and Yang to the unity of Wu Chi. In humans, this hidden force is Yi. Yi is intention and the motivation to action and calmness. Yi is the force which divides Wu Chi into Yin and Yang, and Yi is also the force which combines Yin and Yang into Wu Chi. When this hidden force is applied to natural Chi or energy, it is the EMF (electromagnetic force) which is building up or diminishing. In one word, Tai Chi is the "cause" of Wu Chi and of the division into Yin and Yang.

When Yin and Yang theory is applied to man, its root of action is your Yi (wisdom mind). It is your mind which decides if you will change your Wu Chi state into the Yin and Yang state, or if you will lead yourself from Yin and Yang into Wu Chi. That means that your Yi is the EMF which determines the entire situation: your Yin and Yang strategy, actions, or the Chi movements in Tai Chi Chi Kung.

It is also said: "Tai Chi begets two poles, two poles produce four phases, four phases generate eight trigrams (gates), and eight trigrams initiate sixty-four hexagrams" (Figure 2-1). You can see that even Tai Chi is divided into Yin and Yang, that Yin or Yang themselves are again divided into Yin and Yang, and so on without end. For example, when Yin and Yang are divided in fighting strategy, each one must be subdivided into Yin and Yang, and each Yin and Yang must balance each other. The deeper you can analyze these layers and subdivisions of Yin and Yang and make them balance each other, the deeper you will be able to understand Tai Chi Chuan and Tai Chi Chi Kung.

Next, I would like to point out the basic Yin and Yang concepts in Tai Chi training. I hope this will help to give you a clearer understanding of the essence of Tai Chi, and thereby avoid errors and confusion in your training.

1. **Tai Chi includes: A. Still Meditation (Yin), and B. Moving Meditation (Yang)**(Figure 2-2).

Yin still meditation can strengthen the mind (i.e., the EMF of the Chi), and can build up the Chi to a higher level. The still meditation of Tai Chi Chi Kung can open the paths of the Conception (Yin) and Governing (Yang) Vessels, and increase the Chi stored in them. When the Chi in these two vessels is abundant, the Chi circulating in the twelve primary channels will be abundant, and therefore your physical body will be able to function more efficiently. Developing the Yi and the Chi through still meditation is the root of physical power. Remember: **ONLY WHEN THE CHI IS STRONG CAN THE PHYSICAL BODY MANIFEST POWER. CHI IS THE YIN SIDE OF POWER, WHILE THE PHYSICAL MANIFESTATION IS THE YANG SIDE.**

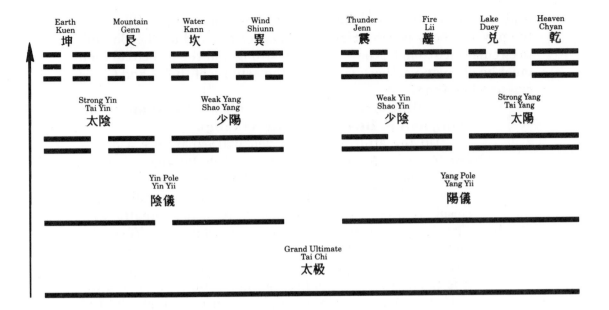

Figure 2-1. The Eight Trigrams are derived from Tai Chi

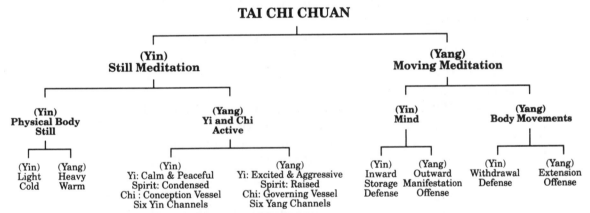

Figure 2-2. The Yin and Yang of Tai Chi

According to this theory, moving meditation is considered Yang because it manifests the Yi and Chi stored by Yin still meditation through the actions of the physical body.

The correct way of martial Tai Chi training is to practice both Yin still meditation and Yang moving physical manifestation equally. Many Tai Chi practitioners today are ignoring the Yin still meditation and practicing only the external moving manifestation. They do not realize that building up the Yi and Chi is the key to effective Chi Kung and martial power (Jing) training.

Still meditation and moving meditation can also be divided into Yin and Yang:

A. Still Meditation includes: a. The Stillness of the Body (Yin), and b. The Activity of the Yi and Chi (Yang).

In still meditation, the physical body should be very still, relaxed, and calm. This opens the Chi channels and allows the Yi to lead the Chi strongly and without any stagnation. This stillness of the physical body is Yin. However, in order to build up the Chi and to circulate it strongly, the Yi must be strong and the Chi circulation must be alive and active. Therefore, the activity of the Yi and Chi is classified as Yang.

a. **The Stillness of the Body includes: i. Light and Cold (Yin), and ii. Heavy and Warm (Yang).**

During still meditation you will experience a different feeling. Normally, when you inhale, your physical body feels light and cold, and when you exhale, you feel heavy and warm. Naturally, all of these symptoms are closely related to the Chi Kung strategy, your breathing.

b. **The Activity of the Yi and Chi includes:** i. the Yi is calm and peaceful, and the spirit is condensed. The Chi is circulating in the Conception Vessel and the six Yin channels, and it is condensing into the marrow and brain (Yin), and ii. the Yi is excited and aggressive, and the spirit is raised. The Chi is circulating in the Governing Vessel and the six Yang channels, and it is expanding to the skin (Yang).

B. **Moving Meditation includes: a. Mind (Yin), and b. Movement (Yang).**

In moving meditation, although the physical movements stimulate the body, the mind should remain calm so that it can lead the Chi smoothly and calmly. Therefore, the motion of the physical body is Yang and the calm mind is Yin.

a. **Mind: i. Chi Condensing for Defense or Jing Storage (Yin), and ii. Chi Expanding for Attack (Yang).**

When your mind is on defending or on storing Jing for an attack, it will lead the Chi inward, the body will feel cold, and the Chi of the body will condense into the marrow. This mind is therefore classified as Yin. This condensing process is usually coordinated with inhalation in the reverse abdominal breathing, and this inhalation is also classified as Yin.

However, when your mind is on an attack, it will lead Chi to the surface of the skin and to the limbs to energize the muscles to a higher level of efficiency. When this happens, the body feels warm and the energy of the body feels like it is expanding. Therefore, it is classified as Yang. Normally, this offensive process is coordinated with exhalation in the reverse abdominal breathing, which is also classified as Yang.

b. **Motion: i. Withdrawal and Defense (Yin), and ii. Expansion and Offense (Yang).**

In the movement of Tai Chi Chuan, the withdrawing and defensive movements are Yin, while the expanding and offense movements are Yang. When you reach the level where the Yi, Chi, and movements are united, you have touched the essence of Tai Chi Chuan.

Naturally, the Yin defensive movements of Tai Chi can again be divided into Yin and Yang. For example, a completely defensive withdrawal movement is a Yin defense, whereas, if the withdrawal is used to set up an offense, it is considered a Yang defense. This is because the Yi stays Yang, even though the movement is Yin.

Similarly, in the Yang expanding, offensive movements, if the offensive movement is purely for striking, then it is Yang. However, if the offensive movement is used to set up for a retreat, the Yi is Yin, so the offensive movement is strategically Yin.

2. Tai Chi Breathing includes: A. Normal Breathing (Yin), and B. Reverse Breathing (Yang)(Figure 2-3).

Breathing is considered the strategy in Chinese Chi Kung. How you coordinate your breathing allows you to regulate your body and lead your Chi efficiently. There are two ways of breathing which are commonly used in Tai Chi. The first way is called "normal abdominal breathing" or "Buddhist breathing," while the other way is called "reverse abdominal breathing" or "Taoist breathing." In normal abdominal breathing, when you inhale the abdomen (or Dan Tien) expands, and when you exhale the abdomen withdraws. However, in reverse abdominal breathing the abdomen (or Dan Tien) withdraws when you inhale, and expands when you exhale. It is usually easier to keep your body relaxed and feeling comfortable with normal abdominal breathing, so that is the method commonly used by those who practice Tai Chi only for health.

As for reverse abdominal breathing, many Tai Chi practitioners today falsely believe that the reverse breathing technique is against the way of the Tao. This is not true. It is simply used for different purposes. Try this simple experiment. Place one hand on your abdomen, and hold the other in front of you as if you were pushing something. Inhale deeply, and as you exhale, imagine that you are pushing a heavy object. You will easily see that, when you try to push as strongly as possible, you automatically use reverse breathing. This is the method which is commonly used in weightlifting

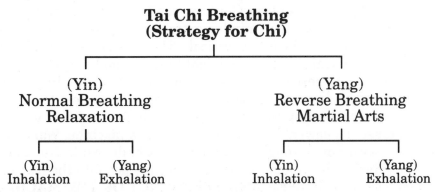

Figure 2-3. The Yin and Yang of Breathing

competition. The competitors often wear a thick belt to support their abdomens and increase their power.

The rationale for reverse breathing is quite simple. You can lead a much stronger flow of Chi to the limbs and manifest more power if you also, simultaneously, direct another flow of Chi to your Dan Tien. This is in accordance with the basic law of physics which states that for every action there must be an equal and opposite reaction. If you are still not convinced, try another experiment. Blow up a balloon, and hold a hand on your abdomen to see how it moves.

You can see from these experiments that reverse breathing is in accord with the Tao. It should be used whenever you need to lead Chi to the limbs to efficiently manifest power, as when you are fighting. Because it expands the Chi and energizes the body it is considered Yang in comparison to normal breathing.

A. Normal Breathing includes: a. Inhalation (Yin), and b. Exhalation (Yang).

In normal breathing, inhalation is classified as Yin because the Chi is led from the limbs to the Dan Tien, and exhalation is Yang because the Chi is led to the limbs.

B. Reverse Breathing includes: a. Inhalation (Yin), and b. Exhalation (Yang).

Similarly, in reverse breathing, inhalation is classified as Yin because the Chi is led from the limbs to the Dan Tien and from the skin to the bone marrow. Naturally, the exhalation is Yang because the Chi is led to the limbs from the Dan Tien and to the skin from the bone marrow.

3. Tai Chi Jing includes: A. Nei Jing (Yin), and B. Wai Jing (Yang); also A. Defensive (Yin), and B. Offensive (Yang).

There are two ways to classify the Yin and Yang of Tai Chi's Jing (power). The first way is according to how the Jing was generated, and the second way is according to the purpose of the Jing.

First, Tai Chi Jing can be classified as Nei Jing (Internal Jing), which is Yin; and Wai Jing (External Jing), which is Yang. Nei Jing training is the critical key which enables the Wai Jing to manifest its maximum power. Nei Jing includes how to build up the Chi to a higher level and how to lead Chi from the Dan Tien to the limbs to energize the muscles. The mind is extremely important in Nei Jing training, and the methods are critical. The master usually does not reveal Nei Jing training to the student until he can be trusted.

Wai Jing concerns the physical movements of the Jing, which include the movement from the root of the stance, how to use the waist to direct the Jing from the legs to the limbs, and how to manifest and use the power. To use the analogy of a machine, Wai Jing is involved with how strongly the machine is built, while Nei Dan is concerned with the amount of energy which is put into the machine. Remember: **THE POWER AND EFFICIENCY OF THE MACHINE IS DETERMINED BY THE ENERGY SUPPLY.**

Next, if we classify Jing according to its purpose, then the defensive Jing (Shoou Jing) is Yin while the offensive Jing (Fa Jing) is Yang. Typical examples of defensive Jing are Listening Jing, Yielding Jing, Leading Jing, and Neutralizing Jing. Typical examples of offensive Jing are Pushing Jing, Striking Jing, Wardoff Jing, etc.

Jing can also be classified according to how it Jing is manifested. For example, Jing which relies more on muscles than Chi is classified as Hard Jing (Yang), while Jing which reduces the use of muscle to a very low level is classified as Soft Jing (Yin). Naturally, like all other cases of Yin and Yang classification, these can be further sub-classified.

4. The Secret of Yin and Yang in Tai Chi practice.

Kan-Lii and Yin-Yang adjustments are critical keys for success in Chi Kung, and so adjusting them is one of the main subjects of both training and research. According to the experience of the last thousand years, a Nei Dan Chi Kung practitioner who wishes to adjust his Kan and Lii efficiently must learn how to regulate his Yi and breathing. There are also several "Chiaw Men" (Tricky Doors) which have usually been kept secret, and only taught when the student had earned the trust of his master. One of the secrets is to touch the tongue to the roof of the mouth. This connects the Yin Conception Vessel to the Yang Governing Vessel. Without this, the Chi could stagnate in the mouth area and make the body too Yang.

Another secret of Nei Dan training is using the Yi and the movement of the Huiyin cavity (Figure 2-4) and the anus. When this is done in coordination with the correct breathing, it can effectively adjust the body's Yin and Yang. It is quite simple. If you use normal breathing, when you inhale and expand your abdomen you also gently expand your Huiyin and anus, and when you exhale and withdraw your abdomen you gently hold your Huiyin and anus up. It is important to know that **HOLDING UP DOES NOT MEAN LIFTING UP OR TENSING. TENSING CAUSES CHI STAGNATION.**

Practicing Tai Chi Chuan with normal breathing relaxes the body and mind and opens the twelve primary channels. This can effectively maintain your health. With normal breathing, when you inhale the Lower Dan Tien expands, you gently expand the Huiyin and anus, and at the same time use your Yi to lead the Chi to the bottom of your feet and further into the ground. However, when you exhale, the Lower Dan Tien withdraws, you gently hold up your Huiyin and anus, and at the same time use your Yi to lead the Chi upward to the Baihui. This is a calming and cleaning process which is used in almost all Chi Kung practices. Normal breathing and the coordination of the Huiyin and anus is the key to calming down both the physical and mental bodies, and it is one of the most effective ways of changing the body from Yang to Yin.

With reverse abdominal breathing you withdraw the abdomen and hold up the Huiyin and anus when you inhale, and expand the abdomen and gently expand your Huiyin and anus when you exhale. This enables you to energize the body and lead Chi out to the skin on the exhale, and lead Chi into the marrow and internal organs on the inhale. The inhale also leads Chi upward to your brain through the inside of your spine. If you do this right you will feel cold and light, and you may also experience a sense of rising. When you exhale this way you should feel hot, expanding, heavy, and sinking. You can see that inhaling is a way to become more Yin, while exhaling is a way to become more Yang. Inhalation is Kan while exhalation is Lii.

In conclusion, when you practice Tai Chi Chi Kung it is important to remember to keep the tip of your tongue touching the center of the roof of your mouth. This must be done lightly, because if you exert too much pressure the tongue muscles will tense and stagnate the Chi circulation. In addition, you must remember that your Huiyin and anus must move up and down in coordination with your breathing. As always, your Yi remains the main key to successful Yin and Yang adjustment. Normal breathing is more effective in leading the Chi up and down, while reverse breathing is more efficient in leading the Chi inward and outward.

5. Others.

There are many other things in Tai Chi which are classified as Yin and Yang, but it would take too many pages to discuss them.

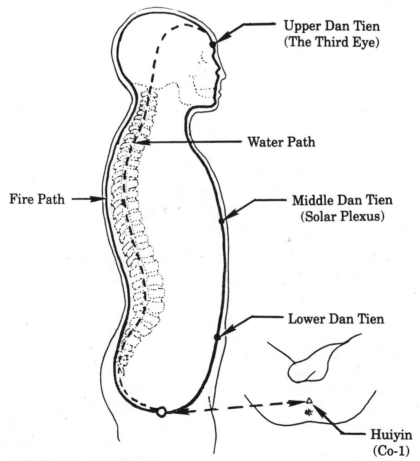

Figure 2-4. The Huiyin cavity

However, we will briefly discuss some typical examples. Once you understand the idea, you should be able to classify almost everything in Tai Chi into Yin and Yang.

A. The root is Yin and the limbs are Yang. In Tai Chi Jing, the power is generated from the legs, directed by the waist, and manifested by the limbs. The root is the origin of the power and is therefore Yin, and the limbs manifest this power and are therefore Yang.

B. Relaxation is Yin and tenseness is Yang. When you relax, your body and mind are calm and the Chi can be led into the organs and marrow. Relaxation is therefore Yin. When you are tense, the muscles are manifesting their strength and the power is demonstrated on the surface of the body, so tenseness is therefore Yang.

C. The center of the palm is Yin while the edge and fingers are Yang. In the palm, Chi is distributed from the Laogong cavity (Figure 2-5) to the edge and to the fingers. Therefore, the center is Yin while the edge is Yang.

D. When the palms are facing up or forward, energy is emitted and so they are Yang. When they are facing toward your body or downward, the energy is conserved and they are Yin.

E. Attack is Yang and defense is Yin. When you attack, the attacking hand is Yang and the rear leg which supports the attack is Yin. Also, if you grab the opponent's hand and pull, then the pulling hand is Yang while the front leg which is supporting the pull is Yin. Remember, Yin is the root, source, and cause of the power, while Yang is the power itself.

Again, every example of Yin and Yang can be subdivided into another Yin and Yang, and so on. The deeper you are able to dig, the more you will understand Tai Chi. This is the way to understand the essence and the root of the Tai Chi Chuan.

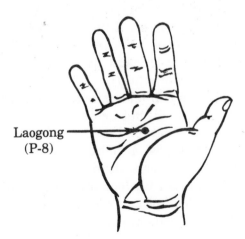

Laogong
(P-8)

Figure 2-5. The Laogong cavity

Chapter 3
Tai Chi Chi Kung

3-1. General Training Concepts

Before we go into the practice of Tai Chi Chi Kung, we would like to point out a few things. First, if you look at your Chi Kung practice as a battle against sickness and aging, then your body is the battlefield, your mind is the general, your breathing is the strategy, your Chi is the soldiers, and your spirit is the morale of the general and soldiers. Therefore, in order to win this battle, you must know your battlefield (body) and learn how to arrange it most advantageously for the battle. The general (mind) who is in charge of the battle must be calm, wise, and always know what he is doing, so that he can set up the best strategy (breathing). When the battlefield, general, and strategy (body, mind, and breathing) are organized correctly, the soldiers (Chi) can be led effectively. You also need good fighting spirit and high morale.

When practicing Chi Kung, you should always pay attention to regulating your body, breathing, and mind. You must keep regulating them until your mind does not have to be on the regulating, and the regulation happens automatically. Then you will be able to feel the Chi, and your Yi will be able to lead it easily and smoothly. Ultimately, you will be able to lead Chi to your head to nourish your brain and raise your spirit of vitality.

Second, although you can learn the theory and movements from this book, the movements will not be as alive and your understanding of them will not be as detailed as if you had learned them from an instructor. In other words, although a book can offer a detailed theoretical discussion which can ultimately lead you to a deep level of understanding, it is often unclear and misleading in its description of movement. A videotape can remedy this lack. However, even if you have both book and videotape, you still will not get the feeling of the exercise. This internal feeling is one of the most important aspects of the exercise that an instructor can convey. However, despite all of these obstacles, thousands of Chi Kung practitioners have reached a high stage of practice through reading, pondering, and training. If you understand the theory, know the movements, and practice patiently and intelligently, then you can gradually accumulate enough experience to achieve a great depth of feeling for the exercise. Only when you have this feeling will you be able to say that you have gained the essence of the training.

Third, remember that theory is the Yin side of knowledge, while practice is the Yang side which manifests the theory. This means that if you really want to understand the exercise, you must both study the theory and practice the exercise. Each one helps the other, so that Yin and Yang can grow together and lead you to the essence of the practice. If you are interested in knowing more about Chi Kung theory, please refer to other YMAA Chi Kung and Tai Chi publications.

In this chapter we will review the keys and the general concepts of successful Chi Kung training. Then we will introduce the warm-up Chi Kung. Beginners frequently ignore the warm-up Chi Kung training. This is unfortunate, because it is almost as important as the Chi Kung practice itself. The warm-ups prepare you by leading your mind and body into a deep meditative state where they are ready for the practice. You will then be able to feel and lead the Chi, which is critical for success. In other words, the warm-up Chi Kung is an integral part of the training.

3-2. Fundamental Training Principles

In this section we will summarize the training principles and rules which we have discussed earlier. During the course of your practice you should always keep them in mind.

Above all, understand what you are aiming for. For example, if you are only a beginner you should first learn to regulate your body until you feel relaxed and comfortable, and then begin regulating your breathing and mind. However, if you have practiced Chi Kung for a while and have already grasped the key points of regulating the body, breathing, and mind, you should then practice using the mind to lead the Chi. Naturally, if you have already reached this level, your target will be learning how to regulate your spirit. The process of regulation is crucial in Chi Kung, so let us review the procedures before we start discussing the actual training.

1. Regulating the Body (Tyau Shenn) 調身

Regulating the body is adjusting your body until it is relaxed, centered, balanced, and rooted. For example, when you practice a pushing movement, the muscles should be relaxed to such a deep level that you can feel your arms relax all the way to the marrow. Only then can the Chi be led into the marrow and also to the surface of the skin. In addition, your movements must be coordinated with the movement of your torso. This enables your whole body to move smoothly and continuously as a unit. The coordination of the body enables you to find your balance. In every movement, your body must be upright (i.e., the head suspended) and rooted, and your pushing arm must also be rooted. For example, in a pushing movement your elbow must be sunk and your shoulder dropped. This allows you to find the root of the push, and makes it possible for your Yi to strongly lead your Chi. You can see that regulating the body is the most important and basic process in any Chi Kung practice.

2. Regulating the Breathing (Tyau Shyi) 調息

When you have reached a level where you feel comfortable and natural and your body is relaxed, centered, rooted, and balanced, then the Chi circulation in your body will not be stagnant. In order to use your mind to lead the Chi efficiently, you must learn to regulate your breathing - which is the strategy of Chi Kung practice. If you breathe correctly, your mind will be able to lead your Chi effortlessly.

There are two common ways of breathing in Chi Kung: "Normal Abdominal Breathing" and "Reverse Abdominal Breathing." Normal Abdominal Breathing is commonly used to lead the Chi to circulate in the primary Chi channels. This helps you to relax both physically and mentally. However, if you wish to lead Chi to the surface of your skin and to the bone marrow, you would normally use Reverse Abdominal Breathing. It is more aggressive, and is therefore emphasized generally by martial Chi Kung practitioners.

Regardless of which breathing method you use, it is important to coordinate your breathing with the movements of your anus and Huiyin cavity. A more detailed discussion of these two breathing methods will be given later in this chapter.

3. Regulating the Mind (Tyau Hsin) 調心

In regulating the mind, you first learn how to bring your mind and attention into your body. This is necessary for feeling the Chi circulation. The first step is learning how to control your emotional mind so that it is calm and peaceful and you can concentrate. Then you can use your Yi to lead your Chi.

4. Regulating the Chi (Tyau Chi) 調氣

Once you have learned how to use your Yi to lead your Chi effectively, then you can start working toward several goals in regulating your Chi. First, you want to make the Chi circulate smoothly and strongly in your body. Second, you want to build up the Chi to a higher level to strengthen your body. Third, you want to lead the Chi to the skin and also to the marrow. This will keep the skin fresh and young, and keep the blood factory (the marrow) functioning fully. Finally, you want to lead the Chi to your head to nourish your brain. It is the center of your whole being, and your health will have a firm root only if your brain is functioning well. If your brain is healthy, you can raise your spirit of vitality, which is the main key to the secret of longevity.

In order to reach these goals, you must first learn how to circulate the Chi in your body without any stagnation. This is possible when all of your concentration is on the Chi circulation, and there is no physical stiffness to make the Chi circulation stagnate. In time, it will feel like your physical body gradually disappears and becomes transparent.

5. Regulating the Spirit (Tyau Shen) 調神

Once you reach the stage of "transparency," you will be able to clearly feel the state of your body's Yin and Yang, and adjust them until you reach the state of Wu Chi (no extremity). When you have grasped this Wu Chi center, you will be able to return your whole spirit to its origin (the state before your birth), your Chi will unite with the Chi of nature, your spirit will unite with the spirit of nature, and you will become one with nature. This is the final goal of enlightenment and Buddhahood.

When you practice, you should also be aware of the following:
1. Do not practice when you are too full or too hungry.
2. Do not practice when you are upset. You will not be able to regulate your mind efficiently and may cause yourself harm, especially if you intend to use your Yi to lead your Chi.
3. Do not drink alcohol before practice. It can excite your emotions and Chi and make them unstable.
4. Do not smoke, since it will affect your lungs and the regulation of your breathing.
5. The best time to practice is just before sunrise. Eat a little bit right after you wake up in the morning, then practice about 30 minutes to one hour. If you would like to practice another time, the best time is two hours after dinner. The second practice in the evening will help you relax before sleep.

To conclude this section, always remember that the final goal of Tai Chi Chi Kung is to be natural. When you regulate your body, breathing, mind, Chi, and spirit, you should practice until the regulation happens naturally and automatically. This is the stage of "regulating without regulating." Only then will you be relaxed and comfortable, and your Chi Kung practice be effective and enjoyable.

3-3. Warm-Up Chi Kung

Before you start your Tai Chi Chuan or Tai Chi Chi Kung practice, you should always loosen up first to warm up your body. This will also prepare you mentally, so that you will get the best results.

In this section we will introduce some of the loosening up and warming up exercises which I have practiced for the last twenty-six years. Naturally, these exercises are only examples, and once you have practiced them and understand their theory and purpose, you may then create other movements which work better for you.

Stretching the Trunk Muscles

Theoretically, the first place that should be stretched and loosened is the trunk muscles, rather than the limbs. The trunk is at the center of the whole body, and it contains the major muscles which control the trunk and also surround the internal organs. When the trunk muscles are tense, the whole body will be tense and the internal organs will be compressed. This causes stagnation of the Chi circulation in the body and especially in the organs. For this reason, the trunk muscles should be stretched and loosened up before the limbs, and before any Chi Kung practice. Remember, people die from failure of the internal organs, rather than problems in the limbs. **THE BEST CHI KUNG PRACTICE IS TO REMOVE CHI STAGNATION AND MAINTAIN SMOOTH CHI CIRCULATION IN THE INTERNAL ORGANS.**

For these reasons, many Chi Kung practices start out with movements that stretch the trunk muscles. For example, in the Standing Eight Pieces of Brocade, the first piece stretches the trunk to loosen up the chest, stomach, and lower abdomen (which are the triple burners in Chinese medicine). In fact, this exercise is adapted from the Standing Eight Pieces of Brocade exercises.

First, interlock your fingers and lift your hands up over your head while imagining that you are pushing upward with your hands and pushing downward with your feet (Figure 3-1). Do not tense your muscles, because this will constrict your body and prevent you from stretching. If you do this stretch correctly, you will feel the muscles in your waist area tensing slightly because they are being pulled simultaneously from the top and the bottom. Next, use you mind to relax even more, and stretch out a little bit more. After you have stretched for about ten seconds, twist your upper body to one side to twist the trunk muscles (Figure 3-2). Stay to the side for three to five seconds, turn your body to face forward and then turn to the other side. Stay there for three to five seconds. Repeat the upper body twisting three times, then tilt your upper body to the side and stay there for about three seconds (Figure 3-3), then tilt to the other side. Next, bend forward and touch your hands to the ground (Figure 3-4) and stay there for three to five seconds. Finally, squat down with your feet flat on the ground to stretch your ankles (Figure 3-5), and then lift your heels up to stretch the toes (Figure 3-6). Repeat the entire process ten times. After you finish, the inside of your body should feel very comfortable and warm.

Warming Up
1. Loosening Up the Torso and Internal Organs

The torso is supported by the spine and the trunk muscles. Once you have stretched your trunk muscles, you can loosen up the torso. This also moves the muscles inside your body around, which moves and relaxes your internal organs. This, in turn, makes it possible for the Chi to circulate smoothly inside your body.

a. Abdomen:

This exercise helps you to regain conscious control of the muscles in your abdomen. The lower Dan Tien is the main residence of your Original Chi. The Chi in your Dan Tien can be led easily only when your abdomen is loose and relaxed. The abdominal exercises are probably the most important of all the internal Chi Kung practices.

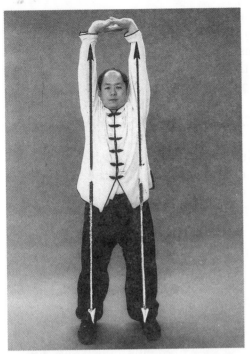

Figure 3-1.

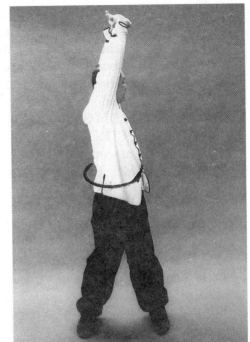

Figure 3-2.

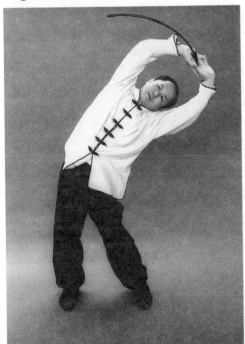

Figure 3-3.

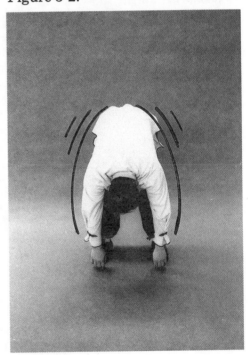

Figure 3-4.

To practice this exercise, squat down in the Horse Stance. Without moving your thighs or upper body, use the waist muscles to move the abdomen around in a horizontal circle (Figure 3-7). Circle in one direction about ten times, and then in the other direction about ten times. If you hold one hand over your Lower Dan Tien and the other on your sacrum you may be able to focus

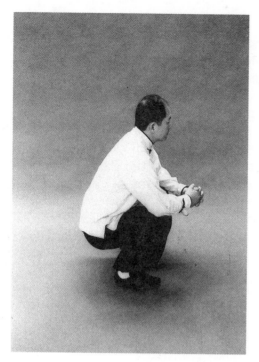

Figure 3-5.

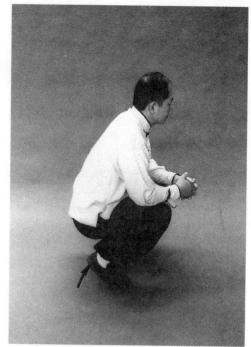

Figure 3-6.

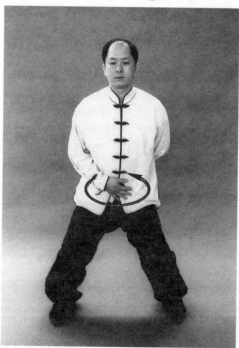

Figure 3-7.

your attention better on the area you want to control.

In the beginning you may have difficulty making your body move the way you want it to, but if you keep practicing you will quickly learn how to do it. Once you can do the movement comfortably, make the circles larger and larger. Naturally, this will cause the muscles to tense somewhat and inhibit the Chi flow, but the more you practice the sooner you will again be able to relax. After you have practiced for a while and can control your waist muscles easily, start making the circles smaller, and also start using your Yi to lead the Chi from the Dan Tien to move in these circles. The final goal is to have only a slight physical movement, but a strong movement of Chi.

There are four major benefits to this abdominal exercise. First, when your Lower Dan Tien area is loose, the Chi can flow in and out easily. This is especially important for martial Tai Chi practitioners, who use the Dan Tien as their main source of Chi. Second, when the abdominal area is loose, the Chi circulation in the large and small intestines will be smooth, and they will be able to absorb nutrients and eliminate waste. If your body does not eliminate effectively, the absorption of nutrients will be hindered, and you may become sick. Third, when the abdominal area is loose, the Chi in the kidneys will circulate smoothly and the Original Essence stored in the kidneys can be converted more efficiently into Chi. In addition, when the kidney area is loosened, the kidney Chi can be led downward and upward to nourish the entire body. Fourth, these exercises eliminate Chi stagnation in the lower back, healing and preventing lower back pain.

b. Diaphragm:

Beneath your diaphragm is your stomach, on its right is your liver, and on its left is your spleen. Once you can comfortably do the movement in your lower abdomen, change the movement from horizontal to vertical, and extend it up to your diaphragm. The easiest way to loosen the area around the diaphragm is to use a wave-like motion between the perineum and the diaphragm (Figure 3-8). You may find it helpful when you practice this to place one hand on your Lower Dan Tien and your other hand above it with the thumb on the solar plexus. Use a forward and backward wave-like motion, flowing up to the diaphragm and down to the perineum and back. Practice ten times.

Next, continue the movement while turning your body slowly to one side and then to the other (Figure 3-9). This will slightly tense the muscles on one side and loosen them on the other, which will massage the internal organs. Repeat ten times.

This exercise loosens the muscles around the stomach, liver, gall bladder, and spleen, and therefore improves the Chi circulation there. It also trains you in using your mind to lead Chi from your Lower Dan Tien upward to the solar plexus area.

c. Chest:

After loosening up the center portion of your body, extend the movement up to your chest. The wave-like movement starts in the abdomen, moves through the stomach and then up to the chest. You may find it easier to feel the movement if you hold one hand on your abdomen and the other lightly touching your chest (Figure 3-

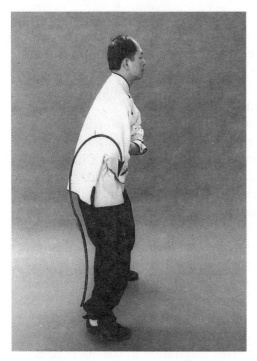

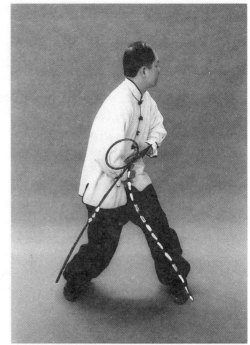

Figure 3-8.

Figure 3-9.

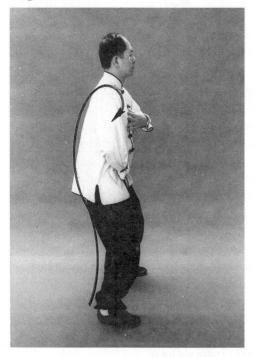

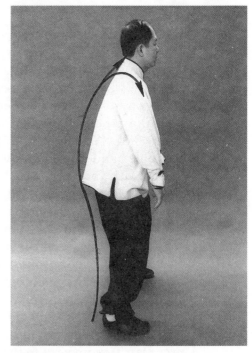

Figure 3-10.

Figure 3-11.

10). After you have done the movement ten times, extend the movement up to your shoulders (Figure 3-11). Inhale when you move your shoulders backward and exhale when you move them forward. The inhalation and exhalation should be as deep as possible, and the entire chest should be very loose. Repeat the motion ten times.

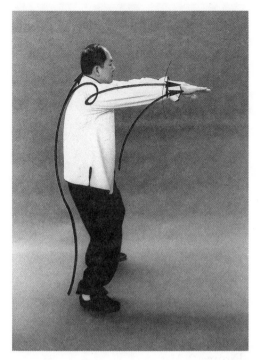 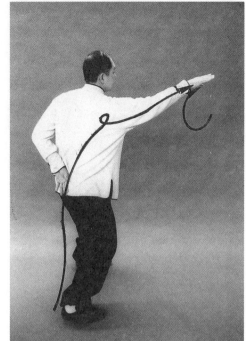

Figure 3-12.   Figure 3-13.

This exercise loosens up the chest and helps to regulate and improve the Chi circulation in the lungs. It also teaches martial Tai Chi practitioners to lead Chi to the shoulders in coordination with the body's movements. In Tai Chi martial applications, Jing (power) is generated by the legs, directed by the waist, and manifested by the hands. In order to do this, your body from the waist to the hands must be soft and connected like a whip. Only then will there be no stagnation to hold back the power. If you are interested in reading more about Tai Chi Jing, please refer to "Advanced Yang Style Tai Chi Chuan, Vol. 1" by Dr. Yang.

d. Arms:

Once you have completed the loosening up of the chest area, extend the motion to your arms and fingers. First practice the motion with both arms ten times, and then do each arm individually ten times. When you extend the movement to the arms you first generate the motion from the legs or the waist, and direct this power upward. It passes through the chest and shoulders, and finally reaches the arms (Figure 3-12). When you practice with one arm, you also twist your body slightly to direct the movement to the arm (Figure 3-13).

These exercises will loosen up every joint in your body from the waist to the fingers. These exercises are in fact the fundamental practice of Jing manifestation in Tai Chi Chuan.

Once you have loosened up your body, you can work on specific areas with special movements. All of the following movements are part of the fundamental training for Tai Chi Chuan. You should

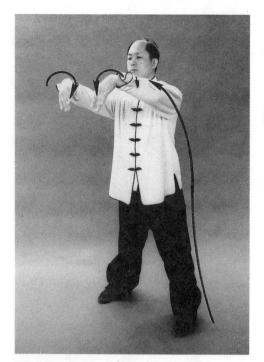 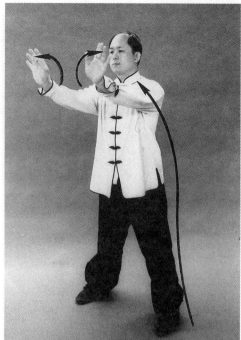

Figure 3-14.   Figure 3-15.

practice each movement until it is smooth and natural and you can feel the Chi starting to flow following the pattern of the movements.

2.   Rotating the Wrists

First, rotate both wrists at the same time. The motion is generated by the legs or waist, moves upward through the chest and arms, and finally reaches the wrists. Hold your arms out in front of you, and rotate both hands first inward ten times (Figure 3-14), and then outward ten times (Figure 3-15). Next, rotate each wrist individually ten times in one direction (Figure 3-16) and then ten times in the other direction (Figure 3-17). Again, the movement is generated from the waist or legs, so that as the wrist turns, the whole body is also moving to generate power for the wrist.

3.   Coiling Forward and Backward

Now extend the motion so that you are coiling your arms. The motion is still generated from the legs or waist, is directed upward and passes through the chest and shoulder, and finally generates the coiling motion of the arms. Start with your hands in front of your chest with the palms facing downward (Figure 3-18), then coil both arms forward (Figure 3-19) and then backward (Figure 3-20). Repeat ten times. Then coil the arms individually. Your right arm coils forward clockwise (Figures 3-21 and 3-22), and backward counterclockwise (Figures 3-23 and 3-24). The left arm coils counterclockwise forward and clockwise back. Exhale with the forward motion, and inhale when coiling your arm back. Do ten repetitions with each arm.

4.   Settling the Wrists

This movement is used frequently in Tai Chi Chuan. Practice first with both hands, and then practice with each hand singly.

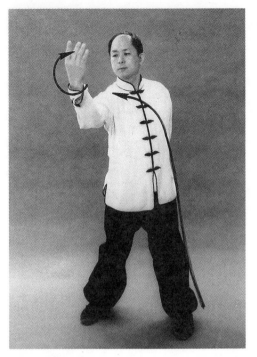

Figure 3-16.

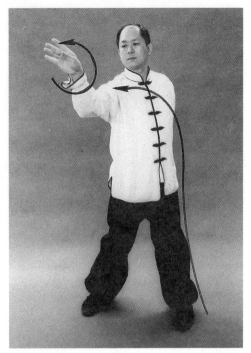

Figure 3-17.

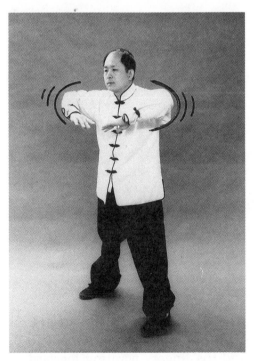

Figure 3-18.

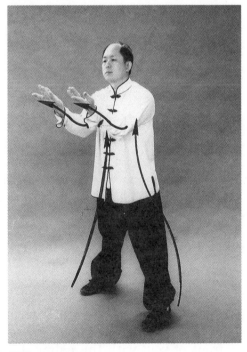

Figure 3-19.

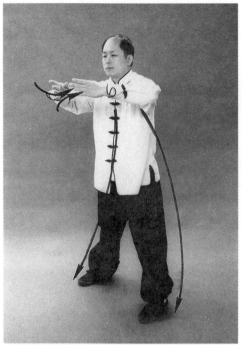

Figure 3-20.

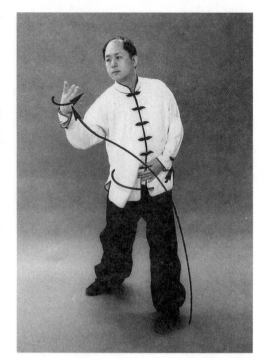

Figure 3-21.

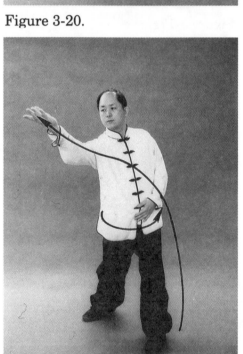

Figure 3-22.

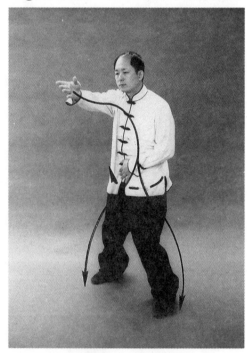

Figure 3-23.

Again, the movement starts with the legs or waist and is directed up to the wrists. To practice using both hands, hold your arms out in front of you, with the palms down and the fingers pointing forward (Figure 3-25). Generate a coiling motion with your legs or waist and, as the motion reaches the hands, lower your wrists so that the palms face forward and the motion becomes a push forward with the palms

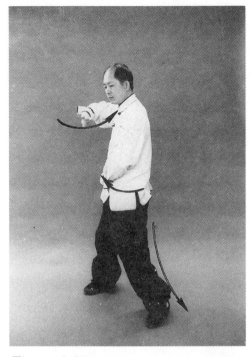

Figure 3-24.

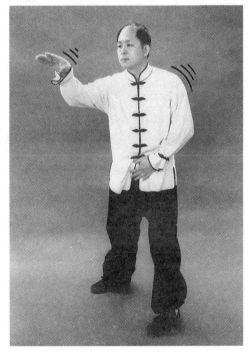

Figure 3-25.

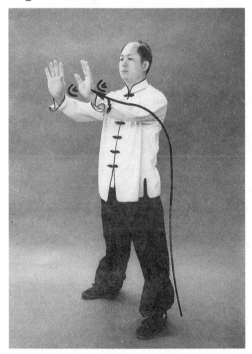

Figure 3-26.

Figure 3-27.

(Figure 3-26). When you practice single handed, you need to twist your body forward and backward slightly so that the pushing power can be directed to the pushing hand more efficiently (Figures 3-27 and 3-28). Practice the two hand press ten times and then each hand singly ten times.

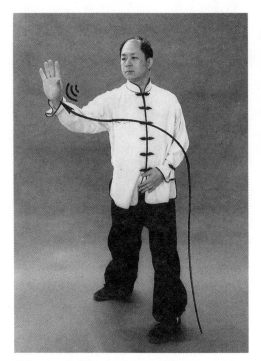 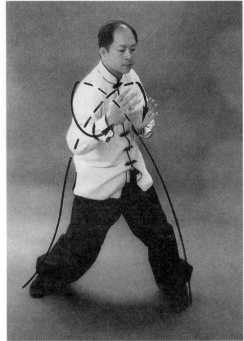

Figure 3-28.   Figure 3-29.

5.   Rotating the Ball

Rotating the ball is one of the most basic exercises to connect your upper body together so that it moves as a unit. Imagine that you are holding a basketball, and rotate it every which way in front of your chest. As always, the motion starts with the legs or waist (Figure 3-29). After rotating the ball about ten times in front of your chest, move the imaginary ball down to in front of your abdomen and rotate it about ten times there (Figure 3-30). There is no fixed pattern for rotating the ball. As long as your arms and body move as a unit and you maintain the sense of holding a ball, you may rotate the ball any way you like. This exercise is an excellent way to thread the entire body together. A more complete explanation and several exercises for Tai Chi ball training will be discussed in the book "The Root of Tai Chi Chuan," which will be published by YMAA at a later date.

6.   Pushing to the Sides

Hold your arms extended to the sides with the fingers pointing to the sides (Figure 3-31). Generate a feeling of motion from the legs or waist and direct it out to the arms. When the motion reaches the hands, settle (lower) your wrists and press to the sides with your palms (Figure 3-32).

Although these exercises are used as warm-ups, if you add your Yi (intention) to each movement you will feel a strong Chi flow. If you are using your Yi to lead your Chi in a relaxed movement, you are already doing Tai Chi Chuan. Remember that these warm-up exercises are offered only as suggestions. They can start you off on the correct path for Tai Chi Chuan or Tai Chi Chi Kung, but once you

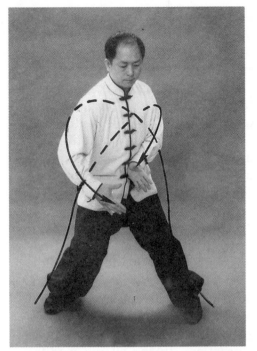

Figure 3-30.

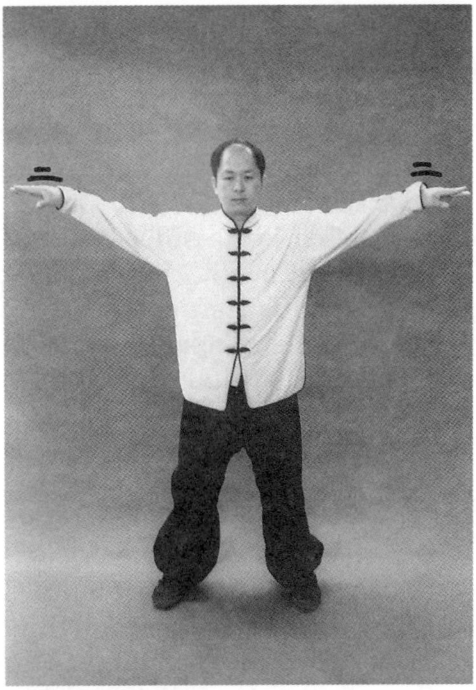

Figure 3-31.

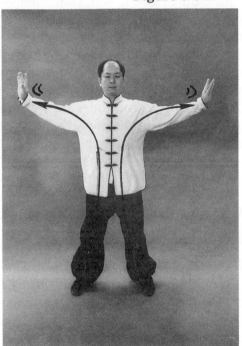

Figure 3-32.

are familiar with them, you may combine them with exercises from other sources or even create exercises of your own.

3-4. Still Tai Chi Chi Kung

Tai Chi Chi Kung can be divided into two parts: the still meditative practice and the moving meditative practice. There are many different sets of moving patterns, each with its own unique purpose and benefits. We will discuss the still meditative practices in this section, and the moving ones in the next section.

Before we start, there are several important concepts which you should understand. As explained in the second chapter, compared with the moving Tai Chi Chuan which is classified as Yang, the still meditation is classified as Yin. Again, in Tai Chi still meditation, the sitting meditation is considered Yin, while the standing still meditation is considered Yang. In both cases the physical body is still, calm, and relaxed as much as possible, and therefore the body is classified as Yin, while the Chi generated and circulated in the Yin body is classified as Yang.

There are a number of other differences between sitting and standing still meditation. First, in the sitting meditation the physical body is relaxed to the maximum, while in the standing meditation the physical body is relatively tensed in certain areas. Second, sitting meditation builds up the Chi through Nei Dan (Internal Elixir) training and completing the Small Circulation (Sheau Jou Tian), while the standing meditation builds up the Chi in the limbs through Wai Dan (External Elixir) practice. In the sitting meditation, the Chi is built up in the Lower Dan Tien, which is the residence of Original Chi. It is located about one to two inches below the navel. The main goal of sitting meditation is to remove all blockages causing stagnation of the Chi flow in the Conception and Governing Vessels. However, the goal of standing still meditation is to build up the Chi by using certain postures which cause tension in specific muscles, energizing them and increasing their level of Chi. Therefore, in the Yin sitting meditation, the body and the mind are both calm, while in the Yang standing meditation, although the mind is calm, the physical body is excited to a degree. If you are interested in learning more about Nei Dan and Wai Dan Chi Kung, you should read the author's book "Chi Kung - Health and Martial Arts."

In this section we will discuss sitting still meditation for the Small Circulation. However, **IF YOU ARE A CHI KUNG BEGINNER, WE RECOMMEND THAT YOU DO NOT START THIS TRAINING ON YOUR OWN NOW**. Nei Dan Chi Kung is hard to understand and experience, especially for Chi Kung beginners. If you do not understand the training theory and practice correctly, you may injure yourself. Wai Dan standing meditation is generally much safer. We are presenting the following discussion for your information, but you should wait until you understand Chi Kung and this training fairly well before you start the practice on your own.

Nei Dan Sitting Meditation

Although Small Circulation is usually achieved through Nei Dan still meditation, there are several Wai Dan techniques which can also be used to achieve the same goal. These Wai Dan Small Circulation practices are normally done by martial artists in the Shaolin styles. For example, some of the Muscle/Tendon Changing

(Yi Gin Ching) exercises are for Small Circulation. This subject is discussed in the book "Muscle/Tendon Changing and Marrow/Brain Washing Chi Kung." There are many Nei Dan techniques for Small Circulation which the different Chi Kung styles have developed. In this book I will only introduce the one which I have practiced.

Small Circulation training has two major goals. The first is to circulate the Chi smoothly in the Conception and Governing Vessels. The second is to fill up the Chi in these two vessels.

We have explained earlier that there are eight vessels in the human body which behave like Chi reservoirs and regulate the Chi level in the twelve primary Chi channels. Among these eight vessels, the Conception Vessel is responsible for the six Yin channels, while the Governing Vessel controls the six Yang channels. In order to regulate the Chi in the twelve primary channels efficiently, the Chi in the vessels must be abundant. Also, the Chi in these two vessels must be able to circulate smoothly. If there is any stagnation of this Chi flow, the vessels will not be able to regulate the Chi in the channels effectively, and the organs will not be able to function normally.

You can see that Small Circulation is the first step in Nei Dan Chi Kung. Small Circulation training will help you to build up a firm foundation for further Nei Dan practices such as Grand Circulation and the Marrow/Brain Washing (Shii Soei Ching).

In order to reach a deep stage of Nei Dan still meditation, it is especially critical that you follow the five important training procedures which we discussed earlier: a. regulating the body, b. regulating the breathing, c. regulating the mind, d. regulating the Chi, and e. regulating the spirit. You also need to know the location of the Dan Tien and the roles which the Conception and Governing Vessels play in Chi Kung. These are discussed in detail in the YMAA Chi Kung book: "The Root of Chinese Chi Kung." It is recommended that you study that book before you start practicing the Small Circulation. Since Nei Dan Small Circulation has been discussed in detail in the earlier YMAA Chi Kung book: "Chi Kung - Health and Martial Arts," we will only review the techniques here.

A.   Abdominal Exercises

You start Small Circulation training by building up Chi at the Lower Dan Tien. This is done through abdominal exercises. You must first learn how to control the abdominal muscles again so that they can expand and withdraw. This exercise is called "Faan Torng" (back to childhood). From birth until about 8 years of age, you move your abdomen in and out in coordination with your breathing. This abdominal movement was necessary for bringing nutrients and oxygen in through the umbilical cord when you were in the womb. However, once you were born, you started taking in food through your mouth and oxygen through your nose, and the abdominal movement gradually diminished. Most adults don't have this abdominal movement when they breathe. The "back to Childhood" exercise helps you to return to this type of breathing.

Once you have regained control of your abdomen, if you continue these exercises you will feel your abdomen getting warm. This indicates that the Chi is accumulating, and is called "Chii Huoo," or "Starting the Fire." These exercises lead the Chi which has been converted from the Original Essence in the kidneys to the Lower Dan Tien, where it resides. The more you practice, the easier this is to do, and the more you can relax your body and feel the Chi.

B.   Breathing

Breathing is considered the "strategy" in Chi Kung. In Small Circulation you may use either Buddhist or Taoist breathing. Buddhist breathing is also called "Jeng Hu Shi" (normal breathing) while Taoist breathing is called "Faan Hu Shi" (reverse breathing). In Buddhist breathing, you expand your abdomen as you inhale and contract it as you exhale. Taoist Breathing is just the reverse (Figure 3-33).

As explained in the last chapter, Buddhist breathing is generally more relaxed than Taoist breathing. Although Taoist breathing is more tense and harder to train, it is more efficient in expanding the Guardian Chi and in martial applications. This point can be clarified if you pay attention to the everyday movements of your abdomen. Normally, if you are relaxed or not doing heavy work, you will notice that you are using Buddhist breathing. However, if you are doing heavy work and exerting a lot of force, for example pushing a car or lifting a heavy box, then you will find that your abdomen tenses and expands when you push or lift (which is Taoist breathing). It is suggested that beginners start with Buddhist breathing. After you have mastered it, you should then practice Taoist breathing. There is no conflict. After you practice for a while, you will find that you can switch from one to the other very easily.

C.   Huiyin and Anus Coordination

After you have practiced the abdominal exercises for about 3-5 weeks, you may feel your abdomen get warmer every time you practice. After continued practice, the abdomen will start to tremble and shake each time you start the fire. This means that Chi has accumulated at the Dan Tien and is about to overflow. At this time you should start to coordinate your breathing and abdominal movement with the movement of your Huiyin (literally "Meet the Yin") cavity and anus to lead the Chi to the tailbone (Weilu cavity).

The technique is very simple. If you are doing the Buddhist breathing, every time you inhale, gently expand your Huiyin and anus, when you exhale you hold them up gently. If you are doing the Taoist breathing, the movement of the Huiyin and anus is reversed: when you inhale you gently hold them up and when you exhale, you gently push them out. This up and down practice with the anus is called "Song Gang" and "Bih Gang" (loosen the anus and close the anus). When you move your Huiyin and anus, you must be relaxed and gentle, and must avoid all tension. If you tense them, the Chi will stagnate there and will not be able to flow smoothly.

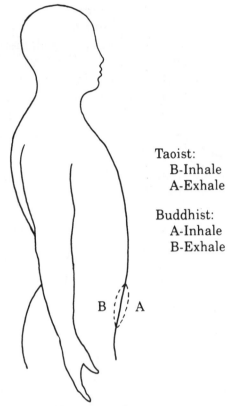

Taoist:
  B-Inhale
  A-Exhale

Buddhist:
  A-Inhale
  B-Exhale

B / A

Figure 3-33. Taoist and Buddhist breathing

The trick of holding up and loosening the Huiyin and anus is extremely important in Nei Dan Chi Kung. It is the first key to changing the body from Yin to Yang and from Yang to Yin. The bottom of your body is where the Conception (Yin) and Governing (Yang) Vessels meet. It is also the key to opening the first gate, which will be discussed next.

D.   The Three Gates

There are three places along the course of the Small Circulation where the Chi is most commonly stagnant. Before you can fill up the Conception and Governing Vessels and circulate Chi smoothly, you must open these three gates, called "San Guan" in Chinese. The three gates are:

a.   Tailbone (Weilu in Chi Kung and Changqiang in acupuncture)(Figure 3-34):

Because there is only a thin layer of muscle on the tailbone, the Chi vessel there is narrow, and can easily be obstructed. Once you have built up a lot of Chi in the Lower Dan Tien and are ready to start circulating it, the tailbone cavity must be open, or the Chi might flow into the legs. Since you are only a beginner, you might not know how to lead the Chi back to its original path. If the Chi stagnates in the legs it could cause problems, perhaps even paralysis of the legs. This danger can be prevented if you sit with your legs crossed during meditation, which will

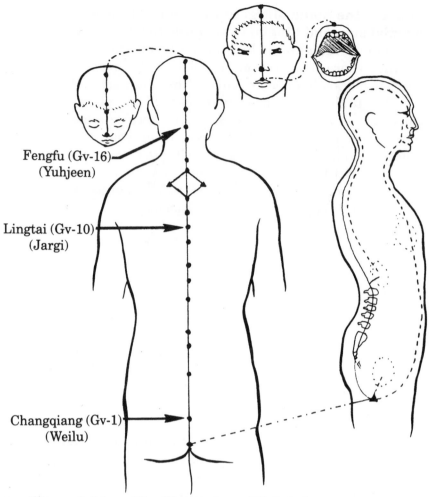

Figure 3-34.　The Changqiang (Weilu), Lingtai (Jargi), and Fengfu (Yuhjeen) cavities

Fengfu (Gv-16)
(Yuhjeen)

Lingtai (Gv-10)
(Jargi)

Changqiang (Gv-1)
(Weilu)

narrow the Chi path from your Dan Tien to the legs and prevent Chi from overflowing downward.

To prevent this kind of problem, you must know one of the important tricks which is called "Yii Yi Yiin Chi"(*1) which means "use your Yi to lead your Chi." Please pay attention to the word "**LEAD**." Chi behaves like water - it can be led, but it cannot be pushed. The more you intend to push Chi, the more you will tense, and the worse the Chi will circulate. Therefore, the trick is to **ALWAYS PLACE YOUR YI AHEAD OF YOUR CHI**. If you can catch this trick, you will find that the Chi can get through the tailbone cavity in just a few days.

Because there are two big sets of muscles in the back beside the Governing Vessel, whenever there is extra Chi flowing through, these muscles will be slightly energized. The area will feel warm and slightly tense. Sometimes the area will feel slightly numb. All of these verify that Chi has been led to that point.

(*1) 以意引氣

b. **Squeeze the Spine (Jargi in Chi Kung, Mingmen in the martial arts, and Lingtai in acupunc-ture)**(Figure 3-34):

The Jargi gate is located between the sixth and seventh thoracic vertebrae, in back of the heart. If the Jargi is blocked and you circulate Chi to it, part of the Chi will flow to the heart and over-stress it. This will generally cause the heart to beat faster. If you become scared and pay attention to the heart, you are using your Yi to lead more Chi to it. This will make the situation worse.

The trick of leading Chi through this cavity is to **NOT** pay attention to your heart, though you should be aware of it. Instead, place your Yi a few inches above the Jargi. Since Chi follows the Yi, the Chi will pass through without too much effort.

You can easily tell when the Chi is passing between the tailbone and the neck, because the muscles will feel numb, tense, or warm.

c. **Jade Pillow (Yuhjeen in Chi Kung and Fengfu in acupuncture)**(Figure 3-34):

The Jade Pillow cavity is the last gate which you must open. The cavity is so named because it is located in that part of your head which rests on the pillow, which the Chinese liked to make out of jade. There is not much muscle in this area, and so the path of the Governing Vessel is narrow, and easily constricted. This lack of muscle creates another problem. Because most of the spine is surrounded by layers of muscle, it is easy to gauge where the Chi is because of the response of the muscles. However, from the Jade Pillow up over the head there is very little muscle, and it is harder to tell what is happening with the Chi. This is especially confusing for beginners, but if you take it easy and proceed carefully, you will soon learn to recognize the new clues. For some people, when the Chi passes through the Jade Pillow cavity it feels like insects walking over their heads. Other people feel numbness or itching.

Be very conscientious when you move Chi through this area. If you do not lead the Chi in the right path, the Chi may spread over your head. If it is not kept near the surface, it may enter your brain and affect your thinking. It is said that this can sometimes even cause permanent damage to the brain.

E. Breathing and Chi Circulation

In Chi Kung, breathing is considered your strategy. Although there is only one goal, there can be many strategies. It is the same as when you are playing chess with someone. Although you both have the same goal, and want to checkmate the other's king, there are many different ways you can go about it. Chinese Chi Kung has developed at least 13 different strategies or methods of training. It is hard to say which is the best breathing strategy. It depends on the individual's understanding, the depth of his Chi Kung practice, and his training goals.

When you train using your breathing to lead the Chi, you should always pay attention to several things. The first is keeping the tip of your tongue touching the roof of your mouth (Figure 3-35). This connects the Yin (Conception) and Yang (Governing) Vessels. This process is called "Da Chyau," which means "building a bridge." This allows the Chi to circulate smoothly between the Yin and Yang vessels. The bridge also causes your mouth to generate saliva, which keeps your throat moist during meditation. The area beneath the tongue where saliva is generated is called Tian Chyr (heavenly pond).

The second thing you need to pay attention to is the strength of your Yi, and how effectively it is leading the Chi. The third thing is how much your Shen is able to follow the breathing strategy. It is said: "Shen Shyi Shiang Yi,"(*2) which means "spirit and breathing mutually rely on each other." As long as the Chi can be led effectively and the Shen can be raised strongly while the body is relaxed and the mind calm, the breathing strategy is being effective.

We would like to recommend several breathing strategies which are commonly used to lead the Chi in training the Small Circulation.

a. Taoist Breathing Strategy:

As discussed earlier, Taoists use reverse breathing, whereby the abdomen draws in as you inhale, and expands as you exhale. This type of breathing reflects and augments the expanding and withdrawing of the Chi. As you exhale, the Chi can be expanded to the skin, the limbs, or even

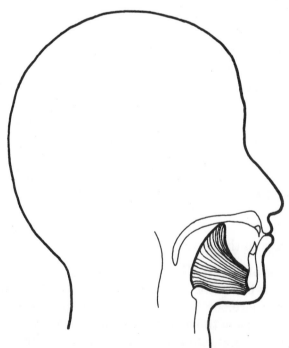

Figure 3-35. Tongue position in Chi Kung practice

(*2). 神息相依

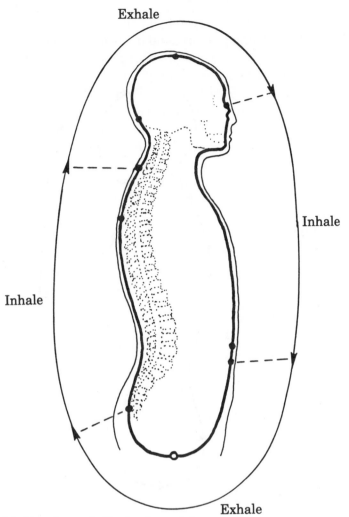

Figure 3-36. Two breath Taoist breathing cycle

beyond the skin, while as you inhale the Chi can be drawn deep into the marrow. Reverse breathing is the natural way your body breathes when you want to get power out. Martial artists use this strategy of exhaling while the abdomen expands. The disadvantage of reverse breathing is that it is harder for beginners. When you do not do reverse breathing correctly, you will feel tension in your abdomen and a buildup of pressure in your solar plexus. This significantly affects the Chi circulation. To avoid this, it is highly recommended that Chi Kung beginners start with Buddhist breathing. Only when breathing this way is easy, natural, and comfortable should you switch to the Taoist reverse breathing.

There are two common ways to use the Taoist breathing to lead the Chi for Small Circulation, one with two inhalations and exhalations per cycle, and the other with one inhalation and exhalation per cycle.

i. Two Breath Cycle (Figure 3-36):

In your first inhale, lead the Chi to the Lower Dan Tien; when you exhale, lead the Chi from the

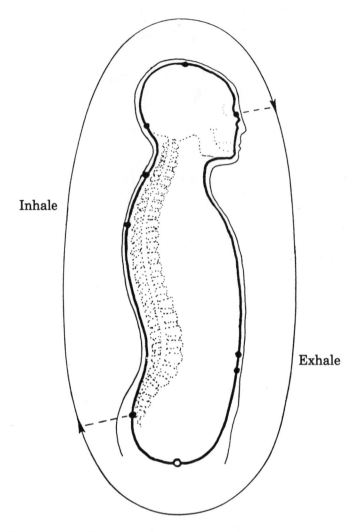

Inhale

Exhale

Figure 3-37. One breath Taoist breathing cycle

Lower Dan Tien to the tailbone. As you inhale again, lead the Chi from the tailbone up along the spine to the level of the shoulders, and as you exhale, lead the Chi over the head to the nose to complete the cycle.

ii. **One Breath Cycle** (Figure 3-37):

On the exhale, lead the Chi from the nose to the tailbone, and on the inhale, lead the Chi from the tailbone to the nose to complete the cycle. In Taoist breathing, the inhalation is always used to lead Chi from the tailbone up the spine. If you try to do this with the exhalation, then you will be pushing the Chi, and not leading it.

b. **Buddhist Breathing Strategy:**

The Buddhists usually use the one breath cycle, but this does not mean you cannot use a two breath cycle. As long as you follow the rules, you can experience many breathing strategies by yourself.

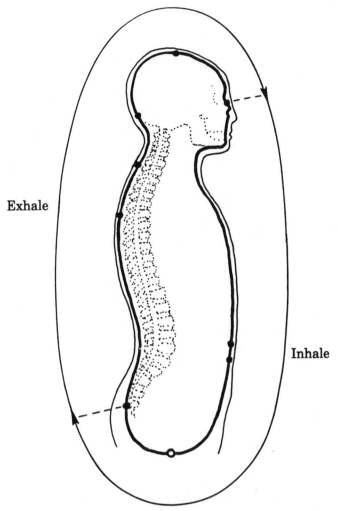

Exhale

Inhale

Figure 3-38. One breath Buddhist breathing cycle

i. One Breath Cycle (Figure 3-38):

When you inhale, your mind leads the Chi from your nose to your tailbone; and when you exhale, it leads the Chi from the tailbone to the nose to complete the cycle.

F. When to Practice

According to the documents, there are three times in the day which are considered best for practice: before midnight, dawn, and after noon (between one and two o'clock). If you cannot meditate three times a day, you should meditate in the morning and evening, and skip the afternoon session.

G. Postures for Practice

When you practice in the morning and in the afternoon, it is recommended that you face the east to absorb the energy from the sun and to coordinate with the rotation of the Earth. For the evening session, you should face South to take advantage of the earth's magnetic field.

When you meditate, you should sit with your legs crossed on a mat or cushion about 3 inches thick. Your tongue should touch the roof of your mouth to connect the Yin and Yang vessels.

Once you have opened up the three gates and circulated the Chi smoothly in the Conception and Governing Vessels, you should then continue meditating to build up the Chi more strongly and to learn to store the Chi in these two reservoirs. Opening up the gates may take only a few months, but building up the Chi to an abundant level may take you many years of continued practice. At this stage, the more you practice, the more Chi you will accumulate. Remember: **ABUNDANT CHI STORAGE IS THE FOUNDATION OF YOUR HEALTH**.

Wai Dan Standing Still Meditation

Over the years, various Tai Chi and Chi Kung masters have created many postures for standing still meditation. Generally speaking, they are safer to practice than the Small Circulation exercises because they build up the Chi locally in parts of the body, rather than directly in the Chi vessels. The ultimate goal of this training is to combine the Chi built up by this Wai Dan practice with the Chi built up in the Dan Tien through the Nei Dan practice. Advanced Tai Chi martial artists will do this during their standing meditation. However, as a beginner you should just do the Wai Dan training, keeping your mind calm and letting the Chi build up naturally through the postures.

We will now introduce two of the postures most commonly practiced by Tai Chi martial artists.

1. **Arcing the Arms (Goong Shoou)** 拱手 **or Embracing the Moon on the Chest (Hwai Jong Baw Yeuh)** 懷中抱月

Stand with one leg rooted on the ground, and the other in front of it with only the toes touching the ground. Both arms are held in front of the chest, forming a horizontal circle, with the fingertips almost touching (Figure 3-39). The tongue should touch the roof of the mouth to connect the Yin and Yang Chi Vessels (Conception and Governing Vessels respectively). The mind should be calm and relaxed and concentrated on the shoulders; breathing should be deep and regular.

When you stand in this posture for about three minutes, your arms and one side of your back should feel sore and warm. Because the arms are held extended, the muscles and nerves are stressed. Chi will build up in this area and heat will be generated. Also, because one leg carries all the weight, the muscles and nerves in that leg and in one side of the back will be tense and will thereby build up Chi. Because this Chi is built up in the shoulders and legs rather than in the Dan Tien, it is considered "local Chi" or "Wai Dan Chi." In order to keep the Chi build-up and the flow in the back balanced, after three minutes change your legs without moving your arms and stand this way for another three minutes. After the six minutes, face forward, put both feet flat on the floor, shoulder-width

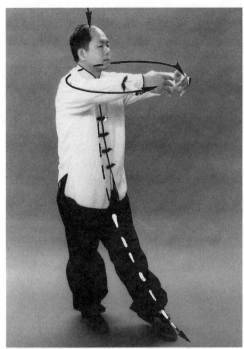

Figure 3-39.

apart, and slowly lower your arms. The accumulated Chi will then flow naturally and strongly into your arms. It is like a dam which, after accumulating a large amount of water, releases it and lets it flow out. At this time, concentrate and calm the mind and look for the feeling of Chi flowing from the shoulders to the palms and finger-tips. Beginners can usually sense this Chi flow, which is typically felt as warmth or a slight numbness.

Naturally, when you hold your arms out you are also slowing the blood circulation, and when you lower your arms the blood will rush down into them. This may confuse you as to whether what you feel is due to Chi or blood. You need to understand several things. First, every living blood cell has to have Chi to keep living. Thus, when you relax after the arcing hands practice, both blood and Chi will come down to the hands. Second, since blood is material and Chi is energy, Chi can flow beyond your body but your blood cannot. Therefore, it is possible for you to test whether the exercise has brought extra Chi to your hands. Place your hands right in front of your face. You should be able to feel a slight sensation, which has to come from the Chi. You can also hold your palms close to each other, or move one hand near the other arm. In addition to a slight feeling of warmth, you may also sense a kind of electric charge which may make the hairs on your arm move. Blood cannot cause these feel-ings, so they have to be symptoms of Chi.

Sometimes Chi is felt on the upper lip. This is because there is a channel (Hand Yangming Large Intestine) which runs over the top of the shoulder to the upper lip (Figure 3-40). However, the Chi feeling is usually stronger in the palms and fingers than in the lip, because there are six Chi channels which pass through the shoulder to end in the

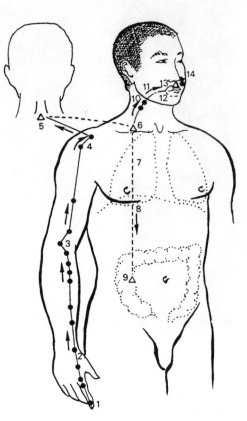

Figure 3-40. The Large Intestine
Channel of Hand-Yang
Brightness

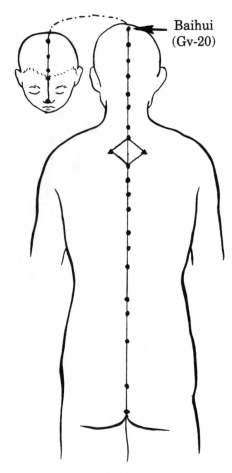

Baihui
(Gv-20)

Figure 3-41. The Baihui cavity

hand, but there is only one channel connecting the lip and shoulder. Once you experience Chi flowing in your arms and shoulders during this exercise, you may also find that you can sense it in your back.

Many advanced Tai Chi practitioners continue to practice this standing still meditation. In addition to building up Chi in the shoulders, they also train using the mind to lead the Chi in coordination with the breathing to complete two Chi circuits. The first Chi circuit is a horizontal one in your arms and chest. On the exhale you lead the Chi to the fingertips of both hands, and then across the gap from each hand to the other. On the inhale you lead the Chi from the fingertips to the center of your chest. The second circuit is a vertical one which connects heaven, man, and earth. On the inhale you take in Chi from nature through your Baihui (Figure 3-41) on the top of your head and lead the Chi downward to the Lower Dan Tien. On the exhale you lead the Chi further downward and out of your body through the Bubbling Well (Yongquan)(Figure 3-42) cavities. When you practice, the two circuits should happen at the same time. If you are a beginner this is not easy to do. If you persevere, however, you will be able to use this exercise as part of your advanced practice.

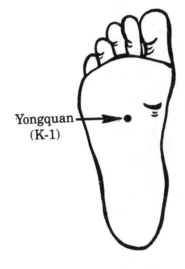

Yongquan (K-1)

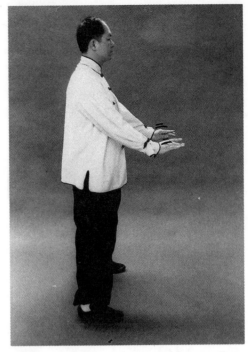

Figure 3-43.

Figure 3-42. The Yongquan cavity

This exercise is one of the most common practices for leading the beginner to experience the flow of Chi, and some Tai Chi styles place great emphasis on it. Similar exercises are also practiced by other styles, such as Ermei Dah Perng Kung.

2. Holding Up the Heaven (Tuo Tian) 托天

This is a very strenuous exercise, so if you are considered old or weak, you should **NOT** practice it. Instead, work with easier and more relaxed moving Chi Kung exercises until someday you feel strong enough to practice this one. Then make sure you start slowly and carefully.

To hold up the heaven, stand with your feet shoulder distance apart, and your arms slightly bent with the palms facing downward (Figure 3-43). Stand still, regulate your mind until it is calm and concentrated, and regulate your breathing until it is natural and smooth. Then, while inhaling, turn your hands to face each other (Figure 3-44) and lift them to shoulder height (Figure 3-45). Then, while exhaling, turn your hands palm downward (Figure 3-46) and lower your body with your palms pressing downward until both of your thighs are horizontal (Figure 3-47). Next, while inhaling, move your arms upward in front of you until the palms are facing the heavens (Figure 3-48). As you raise your hands, follow them with your eyes until you are looking upward. Finally, as you exhale raise your body slightly into the Horse Stance (Figure 3-49). As you stand in this position, breathe regularly and keep your body as relaxed as possible.

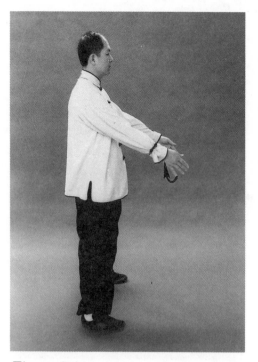

Figure 3-44.

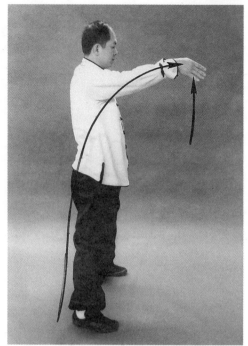

Figure 3-45.

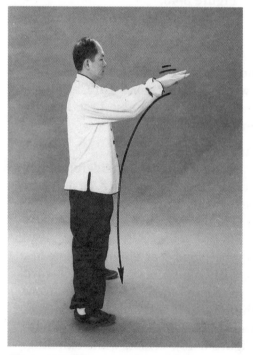

Figure 3-46.

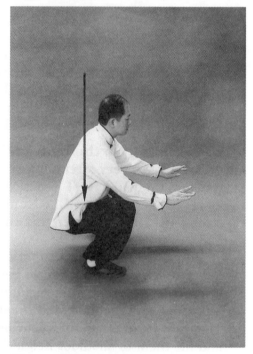

Figure 3-47.

If you are a beginner, only stay in this posture for a minute or so. As you become stronger, extend this time to three to five minutes. Always remember: **YOUR BODY CANNOT BE BUILT UP IN ONE DAY. ADVANCING SLOWLY AND SAFELY IS THE KEY TO SUCCESS.**

As you raise your hands to the final posture, imagine that you are lifting up the heavens, and then stand there as if you were holding up

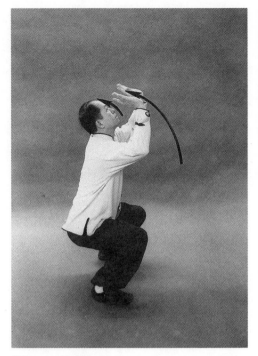
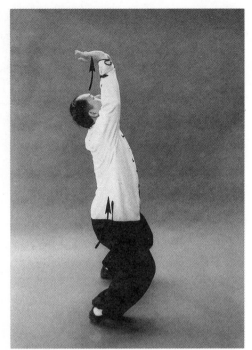

Figure 3-48.   Figure 3-49.

the entire sky. Keeping this idea in your mind will lead Chi from your Lower Dan Tien upward to your hands and also downward to the bottom of your feet. This exercise gradually strengthens your ankles, knees, and hips, as well as the muscles of your trunk and neck.

When you decide to stop, do not just stand up. Keep your arms in position as you inhale and slowly lower your body until both thighs are horizontal (Figure 3-50). Then exhale as you lower your hands to your abdomen (Figure 3-51). Next, inhale and raise your body until you are standing upright, and at the same time lift your arms up to shoulder height with the palms facing each other (Figure 3-52). Finally, exhale and turn your palms downward as you lower them to your waist (Figure 3-53). Stand there for a few minutes and breathe deeply and regularly before moving.

To conclude this section, I would like to remind you that Nei Dan Sitting Small Circulation practice is dangerous for beginners, and you should not start it until you have reached an advanced level. The first Wai Dan Standing Meditation presented here is generally safer for beginners, and Holding Up the Heaven is generally safe for those who are strong enough and in good health. Always remember: **BE CAU-TIOUS AND PROCEED GRADUALLY**.

3-5. Moving Tai Chi Chi Kung

Moving Tai Chi Chi Kung includes both stationary and walking exercises. In this section I will introduce three stationary sets. The first one, which I call the "primary set," is usually used for Tai Chi beginners. I call the second set the "coiling set," since it emphasizes coiling movements. The third set is the "rocking set." It trains the

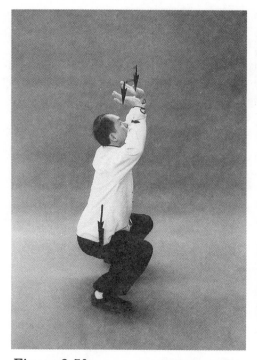

Figure 3-50.

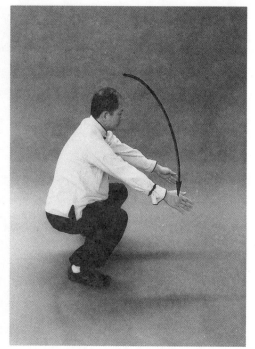

Figure 3-51.

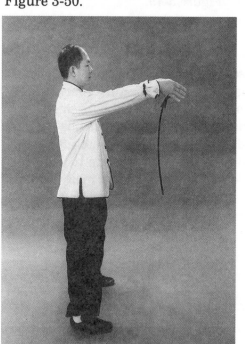

Figure 3-52.

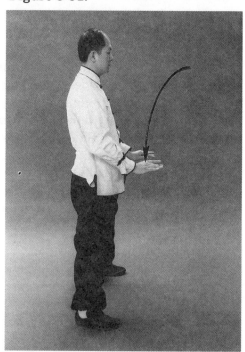

Figure 3-53.

coordination of the hands, feet, and the movement of the body. These three sets actually combine the Tai Chi Chi Kung and the White Crane Chi Kung which I was taught, and they have benefitted not only me but many of my students.

The walking set uses individual movements out of the Tai Chi sequence which are performed repeatedly. The criteria for performing these exercises are exactly the same as for performing the Tai Chi

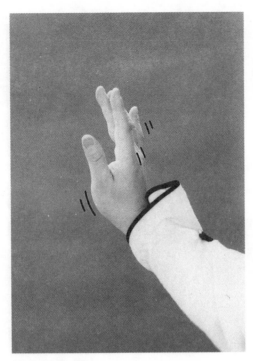

Figure 3-54.

sequence. Since you are doing the same movement over and over again, you do not have to pay so much attention to the form, and can devote all of your attention to regulating your body, breathing, and mind, and to using your Yi to lead your Chi.

Before starting, you should understand that using the proper hand form is another important key to successful training. It is believed that the different hand forms originally came from imitating animals. It was found that holding the hand in the shape of the claw of an eagle, tiger, or crane led the Chi strongly to the hand. The different styles of Tai Chi Chuan have their different ways of forming the hands. It is not surprising that even within the styles some masters use different hand forms, depending upon their personal experience and understanding of Chi. I would like to introduce a hand form which I consider the best for leading Chi to the Laogong cavity in the center of the palm.

In this hand form, which is called "Woa Shoou" (tile hand), the hand is curved like a Chinese roof tile. The thumb and middle finger are stretched forward slightly, and the second and little fingers are pulled back slightly (Figure 3-54). After you hold this hand form for a few minutes you should notice the center of your palm getting warmer and warmer. Use this hand form whenever your palms are open.

Stationary Tai Chi Chi Kung

I. Primary Set
This set of Chi Kung exercises has several purposes:
1. To help the Tai Chi beginner understand and feel Chi. The sooner a beginner is able to understand what Chi is and to feel it, the sooner and more easily he or she can understand the internal energy of the body. This set is simple and very easy to

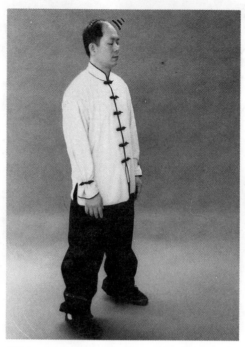

Figure 3-55.

remember, so after a short time you will be able to do it comfortably and automatically, and devote your concentration to your breathing and Chi.

2. To learn how to lead Chi to the limbs. When you have regulated your body, breathing, and mind, you then learn how to lead Chi from the limbs to the Lower Dan Tien when you inhale, and from the Lower Dan Tien to the limbs when you exhale. This trains you in using your Yi to lead the Chi (Yii Yi Yiin Chi), which is very critical in Tai Chi training.

3. To gradually open up the twelve primary Chi channels. After you have practiced this set for a long time, you will find that the Chi is flowing more and more strongly. This stronger Chi circulation will gradually open the twelve Chi channels, and let the Chi circulate more smoothly in your twelve internal organs. This is the key to maintaining good health.

4. To loosen up the internal muscles, especially those around the internal organs. This loosening removes any Chi stagnation near the internal organs, which lets them relax and receive the proper Chi nourishment.

Forms:

1. Stand Still to Regulate the Breathing (Jing Li Tyau Shyi)
静立調息

After you have completed your warm-up Chi Kung, stand still and close your eyes (Figure 3-55). First pay attention to your third eye (Upper Dan Tien), and bring all of your thoughts from outside of your body to the inside. When your mind is calm and concentrated, bring your attention to your breathing. If you are doing only relaxation Chi

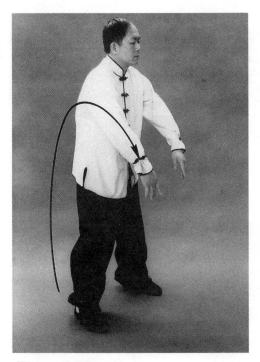
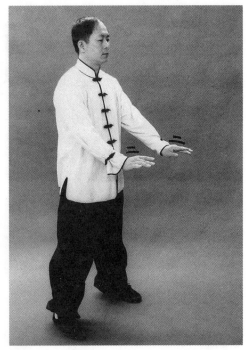

Figure 3-56.   Figure 3-57.

Kung training, use Normal Abdominal Breathing, and if you are training for martial arts, use Reverse Abdominal Breathing. It does not
matter which breathing technique you use, when you withdraw your
abdomen, hold up your Huiyin cavity and anus, and when you expand
your abdomen, relax or slightly expand your Huiyin cavity and anus.
Remember: **DO NOT TENSE OR STRONGLY LIFT UP YOUR
HUIYIN CAVITY AND ANUS.** This will tense the lower part of your
body and stagnate the Chi circulation. After you train this abdominal
anus breathing for a period of time, you will feel that when you
breathe, the lower part of your body is also breathing with you.

2.   Big Python Softens Its Body (Dah Maang Roan Shenn) 大蟒軟身
     After you have regulated your breathing and mind, start moving
your body around slowly. The motion starts at your feet, and flows
upward in a wave through your legs, body, chest, shoulder, arms, and
finally reaches your fingertips (Figure 3-56). The movement feels sort
of like a large snake moving around inside your body. The movement
is comfortable and natural, and there is no stagnation or holding back.
Do the movement for about one to two minutes, until you feel that your
body is soft and comfortable from deep inside the internal organs to
your limbs. After you have finished, hold your hands in front of your
waist with the palms facing down (Figure 3-57). Continue to keep your
mind calm, and breathe smoothly.

3.   The Chi is Sunk to the Dan Tien (Chi Chern Dan Tien) 氣沉丹田
     In this third exercise you are using your mind to lead the Chi to
sink to the Lower Dan Tien in coordination with the movements.
First, inhale and turn your palms towards each other (Figure 3-58)

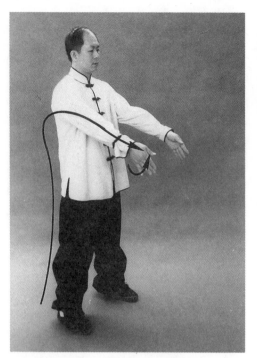

Figure 3-58.

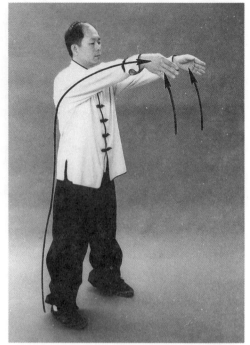

Figure 3-59.

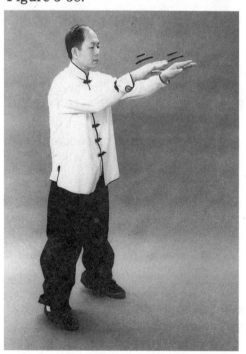

Figure 3-60.

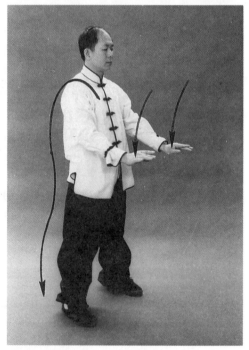

Figure 3-61.

and lift them to shoulder height (Figure 3-59). Then turn both palms downward (Figure 3-60) and lower them to waist level while exhaling (Figure 3-61). Do ten repetitions, and each time you lower your hands imagine that you are pressing something down, and use the mind to lead the Chi to the Lower Dan Tien. Remember, even though it looks like you are moving only your hands, with practice you will be able to generate the movement from your legs or waist.

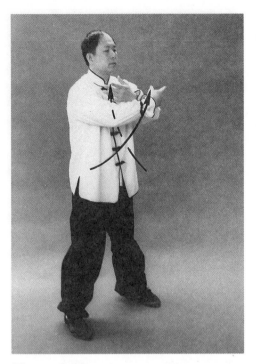 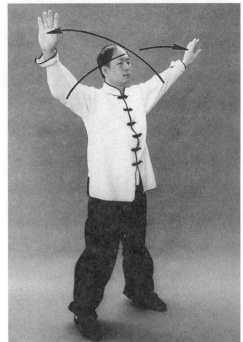

Figure 3-62.   Figure 3-63.

4. Expand the Chest to Clean the Body (Jaan Shiong Jing Shenn) 展胸淨身

After you have completed the last exercise, start circling your arms up in front of you and out to the sides. As they rise in front of your chest they cross (Figure 3-62), then separate up and out to the sides (Figure 3-63). Inhale deeply as they rise, and exhale as they sink out and to the sides. The Yi and the movement start at the waist and are passed to the limbs. The chest area is especially important in this exercise. The deep breathing and the movement of the arms loosens the muscles around the lungs. While doing this exercise you should also visualize that you are expelling the dirty Chi and air from your body and lungs, and pushing them away from your body. Repeat the movements ten times.

5. Pour the Chi into the Baihui (Baihui Guann Chi) 百會貫氣

After you have cleaned your body, you now visualize that you are taking in Chi from the heavens through your Baihui and pushing it down through your chest to the Lower Dan Tien and finally through the bottoms of your feet into the ground. The motion of this exercise is simply the reverse of the previous one. Again, the relaxation of the chest is very important. When you inhale, open your arms out in front of your abdomen (Figure 3-64), and circle them up until they are above your head (Figure 3-65). As you exhale, lower your hands palms down in front of your body while visualizing that you are pushing the Chi downward until it is below your feet (Figure 3-66). Repeat the movement ten times.

6. Left and Right to Push the Mountains (Tzuoo Yow Tuei Shan) 左右推山

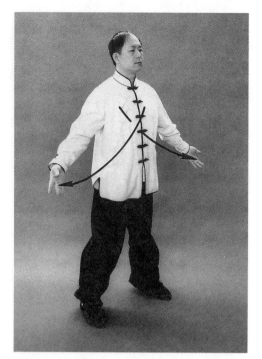

Figure 3-64.

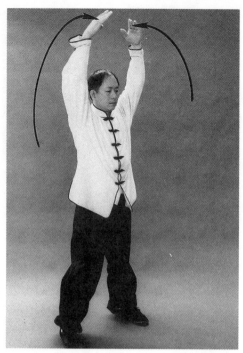

Figure 3-65.

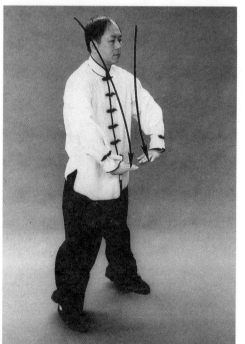

Figure 3-66.

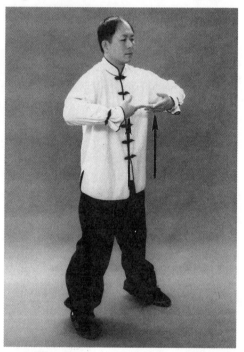

Figure 3-67.

After you have cleaned your body and absorbed Chi from heaven, you start building Chi internally and using it for training. As you inhale, raise your hands to chest height (Figure 3-67). Lower your elbows and turn your hands until the fingers are pointing to the sides and the palms are facing down (Figure 3-68). Keep your wrists loose. As you exhale, extend your arms to the sides. When the arms are halfway extended, settle (lower) your wrists and push sideways with

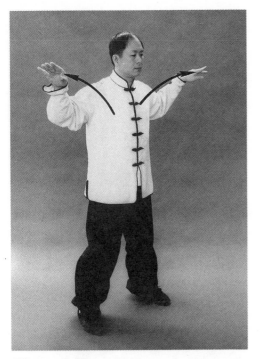

Figure 3-68.

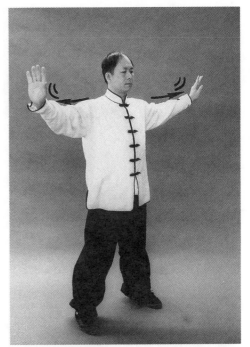

Figure 3-69.

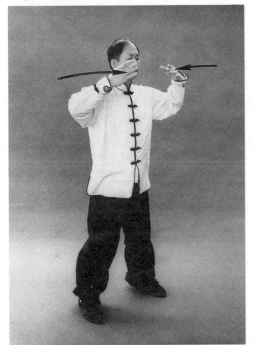

Figure 3-70.

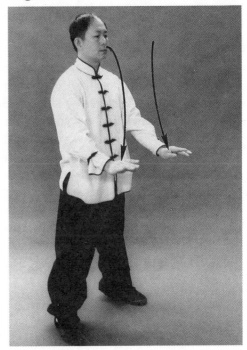

Figure 3-71.

the palms as if you were pushing two mountains away (Figure 3-69). Inhale and bring your hands back with the palms facing inward (Figure 3-70), then exhale and lower the hands in front of you with the palms down and the fingers pointing forward (Figure 3-71). The muscles should remain relaxed throughout the exercise. Do not extend your arms to the sides as far as they can go, because this causes muscle tension and Chi stagnation. Repeat the movement ten times.

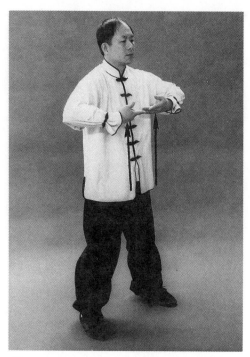 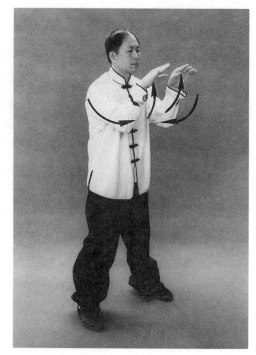

Figure 3-72.   Figure 3-73.

7. Settle the Wrists and Push the Palms (Tzuoh Wann Tuei Jaang) 坐腕推掌

This exercise continues the training of using your Yi to lead your Chi, only now you are pushing forward instead of to the sides. In order to lead the Chi forward to your palms, pretend that you are pushing a car or some other heavy object. Start by raising your arms in front of you while inhaling, as you did in the previous exercise (Figure 3-72). Then lower your elbows and turn your palms forward and downward (Figure 3-73). The wrists are relaxed and the fingers are pointing forward. Exhale and extend your arms. When they are more than halfway out, settle (lower) the wrists and push the palms forward (Figure 3-74). Do not extend your arms all the way, because that would tense the muscles and cause stagnation of the Chi circulation. Next, inhale and draw your hands back, with the palms facing your chest (Figure 3-75), and then exhale and lower your hands to your abdomen (Figure 3-76). Repeat the movement ten times.

8. Large Bear Swimming in the Water (Dah Shyong You Shoei) 大熊游水

When you have finished the last exercise and your hands are in front of your abdomen, raise them again while inhaling (Figure 3-77), then exhale and extend your arms forward with the palms up (Figure 3-78). Inhale and move your arms out and to the sides, turning the palms down, then circle the hands to your waist as you rotate the palms upward (Figures 3-79 and 3-80). Continue by exhaling and extending your arms forward. The motion is similar to the breast stroke in swimming. As always in Tai Chi, the movement is generated from the legs and directed upward to the hands. Repeat the movement ten times.

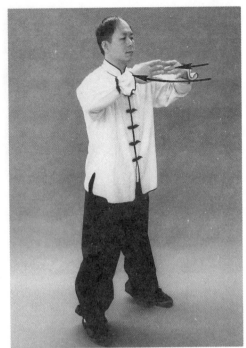

Figure 3-74.

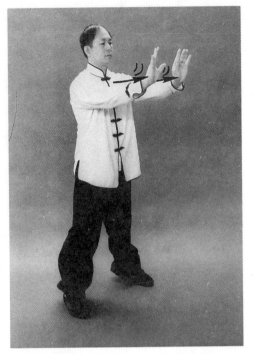

Figure 3-75.

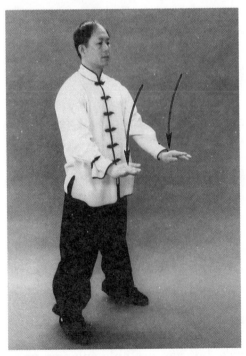

Figure 3-76.

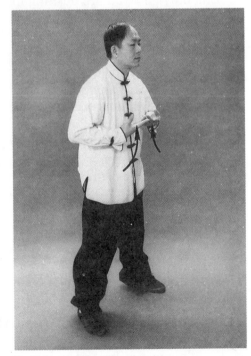

Figure 3-77.

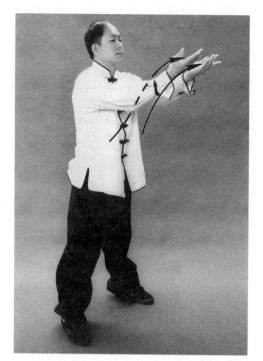

Figure 3-78.

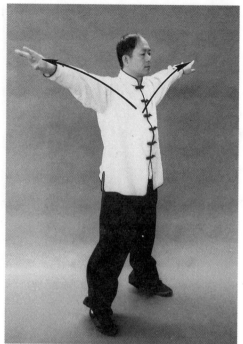

Figure 3-79.

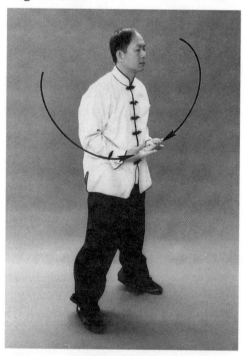

Figure 3-80.

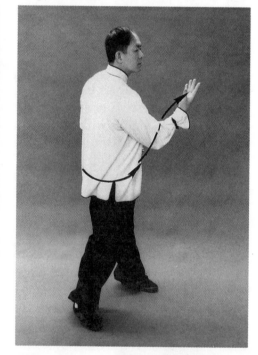

Figure 3-81.

9. Left and Right to Open the Mountain (Tzuoo Yow Kai Shan) 左右開山

This is similar to the last exercise, but you use only one arm at a time. Extend your right arm while exhaling (Figure 3-81), then inhale and turn the palm down as you move it out and to the side (Figure 3-82) and then circle it down to your waist as you rotate the

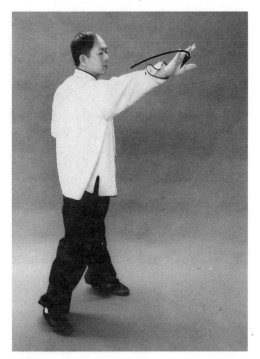 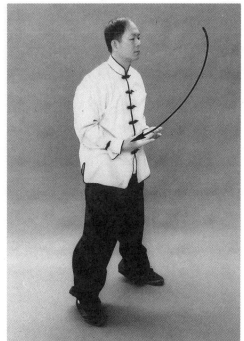

Figure 3-82.   Figure 3-83.

palm upward (Figure 3-83). When the right hand reaches your
waist, do the same movement with the left hand. Do ten repetitions
of the complete movement. Let your chest open and close in coordination with the arm movement, and also turn your body slightly.

10. Eagle Attacks its Prey (Lao Ing Pu Shyr) 老鷹撲食

This exercise uses the reverse of the movement of the eighth
exercise. Starting with your hands at your waist, inhale and spread
your arms out to the sides (Figure 3-84), then exhale as your arms
circle out and forward with the palms facing down (Figure 3-85).
Finally, pull your hands back to your waist as the palms rotate
upward (Figure 3-86). Exhale as your arms move forward, and
inhale as they move back. Again, the motion originates with the
legs. Repeat ten times.

11. Lion Rotates the Ball (Shy Tzu Goong Chyou) 獅子拱球

This exercise is similar to the preceding one, except that you
use only one arm at a time. Starting with your hands at your
waist (Figure 3-87) extend your right arm to the side and then
forward in a counterclockwise movement, turning the palm down
as it moves (Figure 3-88). Then inhale and draw your arm back
to your waist, rotating the palm upward (Figure 3-89). Then
repeat the same motion with the left hand, moving it in a clockwise circle. The movement is generated by the legs, and you can
vary the size of the circles. The most important point of the training is feeling that your body is connected together from the
bottom of your feet to the tips of your fingers. Repeat the complete movement ten times.

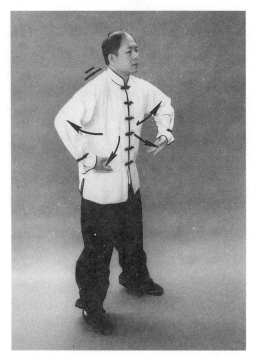

Figure 3-84.

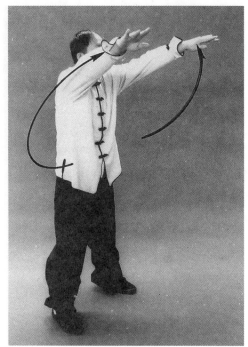

Figure 3-85.

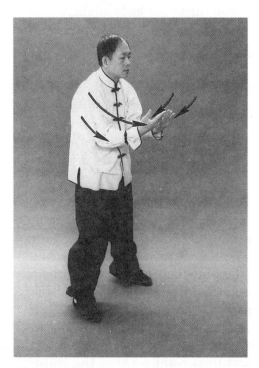

Figure 3-86.

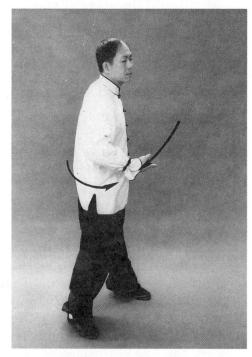

Figure 3-87.

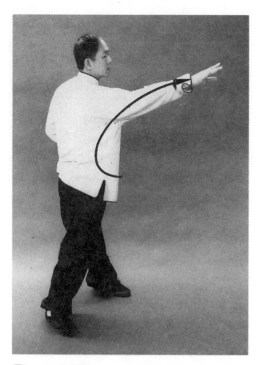 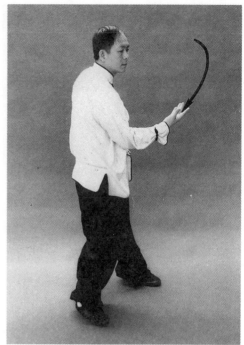

Figure 3-88.   Figure 3-89.

12. White Crane Spreads Its Wing (Bair Heh Liang Chyh) 白鶴亮翅

This last form is used for recovery. In it the arms expand diagonally. When this motion is done in coordination with the breathing, the internal organs will relax and loosen, and any Chi which may still be stagnant internally will be led to the surface of your body. Continuing from the previous exercise, cross both arms in front of your chest (Figure 3-90), then exhale and extend your arms out diagonally, with the right arm up and left arm down (Figure 3-91). Inhale as you draw both arms in and cross them in front of your chest, then exhale and extend them out diagonally again, now with the left hand up and the right hand down. The mind should remain calm and the entire body should be loose. Repeat the entire movement ten times. When you are finished, inhale and move both hands to in front of your chest (Figure 3-92), then turn both palms down (Figure 3-93). Exhale and lower your hands with the feeling that you are pushing something down, and lead the Chi back to your Lower Dan Tien (Figure 3-94). Finally, drop both hands naturally to your sides (Figure 3-95). Inhale and exhale naturally ten times and feel the Chi distributing itself in your body, especially in your hands.

Because you have been standing still for a while, your circulation may have become stagnant and Chi and blood may have accumulated in your feet. You will notice this as a sensation of heat in your feet. Before you move, release the stagnation by rocking back on your heels and raising the front of your feet as you exhale (Figure 3-96), and then rocking forward onto your toes while inhaling (Figure 3-97). Repeat ten times before you start moving around.

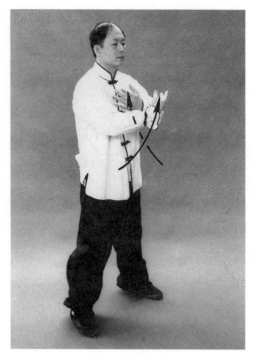

Figure 3-90.

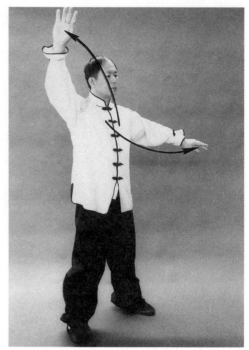

Figure 3-91.

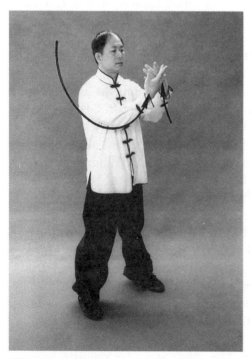

Figure 3-92.

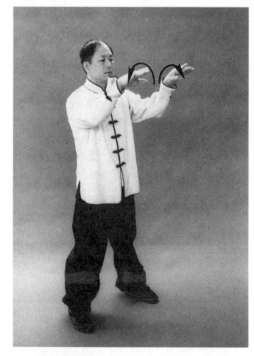

Figure 3-93.

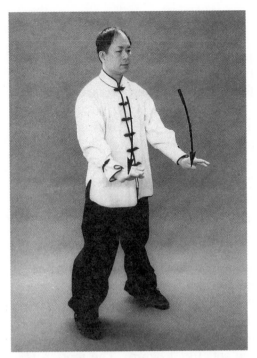

Figure 3-94.

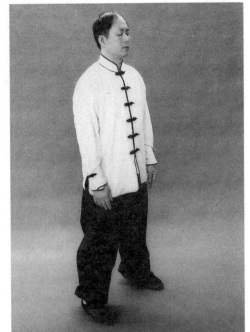

Figure 3-95.

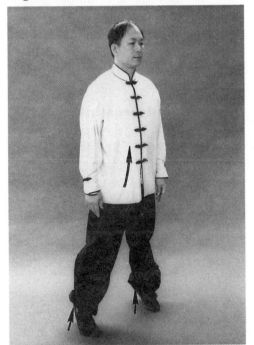

Figure 3-96.

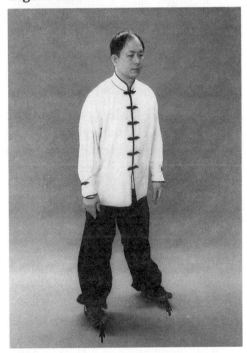

Figure 3-97.

II. Coiling Set

The main purpose of this set is to lead Chi to the surface of the skin and into the bone marrow through the use of breathing and the coiling motion. The principle behind this set is that when a muscle is twisted in one direction and then brought back to its starting position, the muscle is tensed and then relaxed. This continuous coiling motion causes the Chi in the primary Chi channels to be led outward to the surface of the skin and also to be condensed into the bone marrow. This strengthens the Chi which protects your body from negative outside influences, and also keeps the marrow functioning properly.

This coiling set is designed for those who wish to strengthen their Guardian Chi (Wey Chi) and to increase the sensitivity of their "Skin Listening" Jing, which is required for Tai Chi Pushing Hands. You can see that reverse breathing would be more effective than regular breathing in this set, because you can use the exhale to help lead Chi to the skin, and the inhale to help lead Chi to the marrow.

Even though this set was originally designed for martial arts Chi training, it is also a very effective health exercise. An abundant supply of Chi to the bone marrow is the key to health and longevity.

The most important key to this training is concentration. It is the mind which leads Chi to the skin and to the bone marrow in coordination with the coiling motion, so once you are familiar with the movements you should practice leading your mind into a deeper meditative state which allows you to feel or sense the Chi deep in the bones. Every coiling motion should be generated from the legs and directed to the limbs. The entire body should be soft like a whip. The motion is continuous and without stagnation, like the movement of an octopus. Naturally, breathing (which is the strategy of Chi Kung training) is another key to success. Your breathing should be slow, deep, and long, and you should not hold your breath. An additional key to successful training is the coordination of the anus and the Huiyin cavity, which will help your mind to lead your Chi more efficiently.

1. **Stand Calmly to Regulate the Hsin and Breathing (Jing Tyau Hsin Shyi)** 靜調心息

Stand still, with your legs shoulder-width apart and your arms dropped naturally at your sides (Figure 3-98). Both your physical and your mental bodies are relaxed, centered, and balanced. The mind is calm and peaceful. Inhale and exhale smoothly and naturally about ten times in coordination with the holding up and relaxing of your anus and Huiyin cavity.

2. **White Crane Relaxes Its Wings (Bair Heh Doou Chyh)** 白鶴抖翅

Inhale and turn your palms to the rear while rounding the shoulders forward and slightly arcing in your chest (Figure 3-99). As you inhale, hold up your anus and Huiyin cavity. Next, exhale as you turn your palms forward. As you do this, draw your shoulders back and relax your anus and Huiyin cavity (Figure 3-100). Remember, in all of these movements both the Yi and the actual action begin in the feet, pass through the chest, and finally reach the fingertips. Repeat the movement ten times.

3. **Drill Forward and Pull Back (Chyan Tzuann Hou Ba)** 前鑽後拔

Inhale and lift your hands up to mid-chest height. Your chest should be slightly arced in, and your fingers and arms should be in a straight line (Figure 3-101). Pull in the elbows and extend your

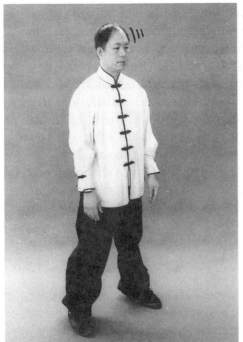

Figure 3-98.

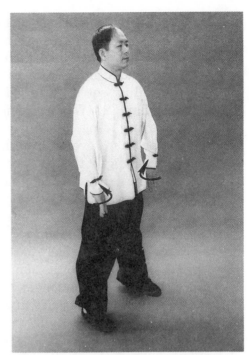

Figure 3-99.

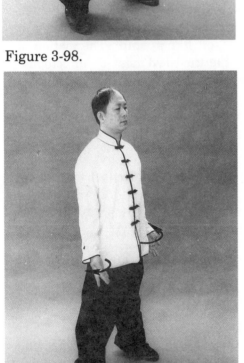

Figure 3-100.

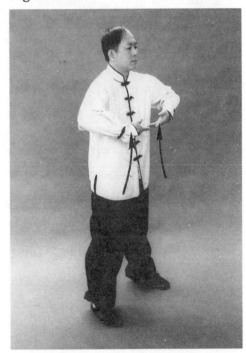

Figure 3-101.

arms in front of you, palm up, as you exhale and gently round your shoulders forward (Figure 3-102). Inhale as you spread your elbows out to the sides and draw your arms back to your chest. Rotate your arms as they move so that they end up with the palms facing your chest. The arms and fingers should be in a straight line (Figure 3-103). As you exhale, press your hands down while keeping them in line (Figure 3-104). Repeat the entire movement ten times.

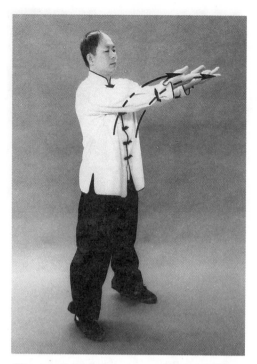

Figure 3-102.

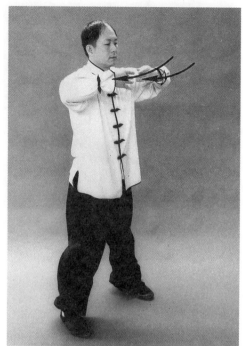

Figure 3-103.

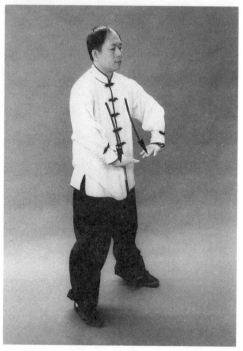

Figure 3-104.

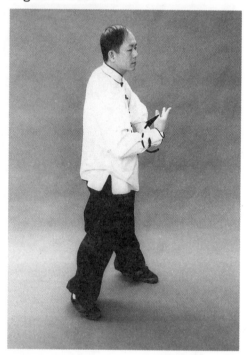

Figure 3-105.

4.　Left and Right Yin and Yang (Tzuoo Yow Yin Yang)　左右陰陽

Continuing from the last exercise, once your hands are in front of your abdomen, drill your right hand forward and rotate the palm upward while exhaling and turning your body slightly (Figures 3-105 and 3-106). Then inhale and pull your right hand back to the original position (Figure 3-107). Then exhale and drill your left hand forward

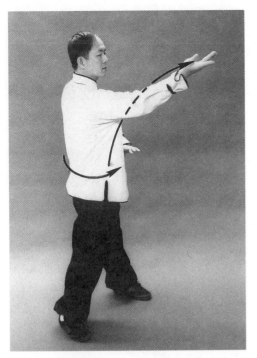

Figure 3-106.

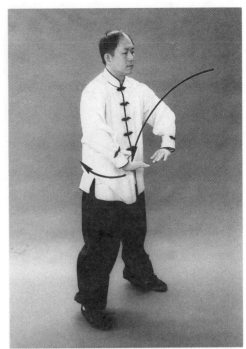

Figure 3-107.

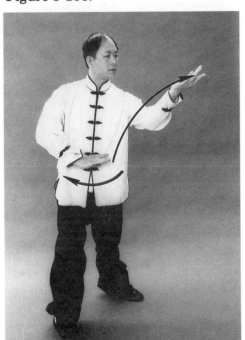

Figure 3-108.

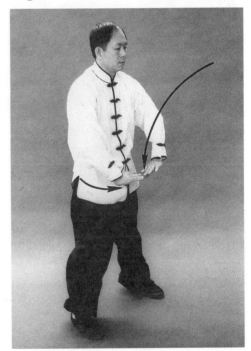

Figure 3-109.

and rotate the palm upward while exhaling and turning your body slightly (Figure 3-108). Do ten repetitions, and finish with your arms lined up in front of your abdomen (Figure 3-109).

5.   Water and Fire Mutually Interact (Kan Lii Jiau Gow) 坎離交媾
    Continuing from the last exercise, inhale, turn the palms up (Figure 3-110) and raise the hands to chest height as if you were

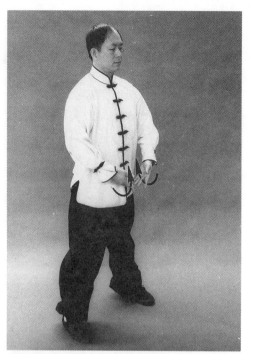

Figure 3-110.

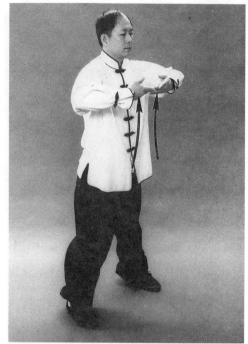

Figure 3-111.

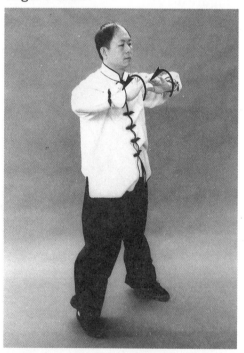

Figure 3-112.

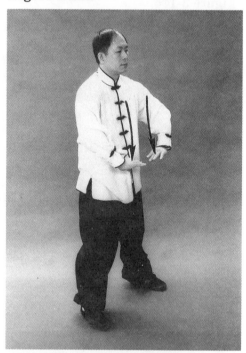

Figure 3-113.

lifting something (Figure 3-111). Turn your palms down (Figure 3-112) and then push them downward to your abdomen, keeping the hands lined up (Figure 3-113). Repeat ten times.

6. Large Bear Encircles the Moon (Dah Shyong Goong Yeuh) 大熊拱月

Continuing from the last exercise, inhale and lift your hands to your chest while turning the palms up (Figure 3-114). As you exhale,

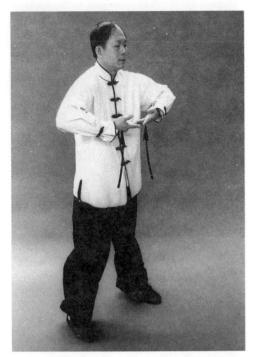

Figure 3-114.

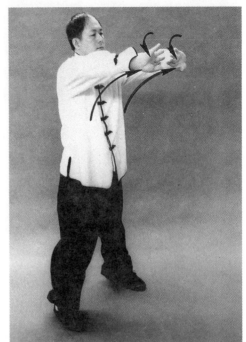

Figure 3-115.

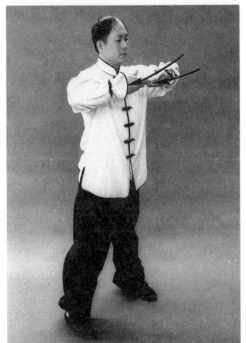

Figure 3-116.

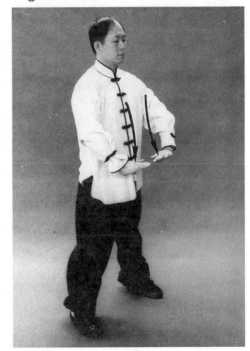

Figure 3-117.

extend and rotate your arms forward so that your arms and chest form a large circle with the palms facing forward (Figure 3-115). As you inhale, move your hands back to in front of your chest, rotating the arms until the palms are facing upward (Figure 3-116). Finally, exhale and push both palms down to your abdomen, keeping both hands in a line (Figure 3-117). Do ten repetitions. Remember, when

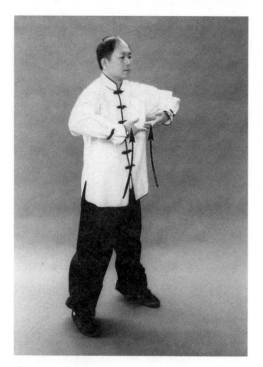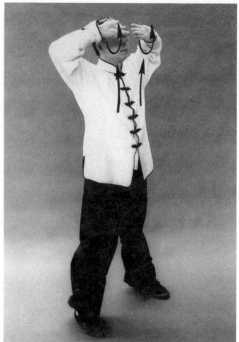

Figure 3-118.   Figure 3-119.

you raise your hands, to imagine that you are lifting something, and when you push down, to imagine that you are pushing something down. Also remember that when you extend your arms they should form a circle with your chest.

7.   Living Buddha Holds Up the Heavens (Hwo For Tuo Tian) 活佛托天

This exercise is similar to the last one, except that now you push your hands upward instead of forward. On the first inhale raise your hands to chest level (Figure 3-118), and then turn the palms upward (Figure 3-119) as you push upward and exhale (Figure 3-120). On the second inhale, rotate your palms and lower your hands to your chest (Figure 3-121), and as you exhale, push your hands palm downward to your abdomen (Figure 3-122). Repeat ten times.

8.   Turn Heaven and Earth in Front of your Body (Shang Shiah Chyan Kuen) 上下乾坤

First turn your palms upward and raise both hands to your chest while inhaling, then exhale and push up with one hand and down with the other (Figures 3-123 and 3-124). As you inhale, bring both hands to your chest (Figure 3-125), and then exhale and push up and down with the opposite hands (Figure 3-126). Repeat ten times.

9.   Golden Rooster Twists Its Wings (Jin Ji Aw Chyh) 錦鷄拗翅

This exercise is very similar to the last one, except that the hand pushing down is behind you. As you inhale, bring both hands to your chest (Figure 3-127), and as you exhale, separate them and push them up and down (Figure 3-128). Then inhale again and bring both hands to your chest (Figure 3-129), separate them, and push them up and down as you exhale (Figure 3-130). Repeat ten times.

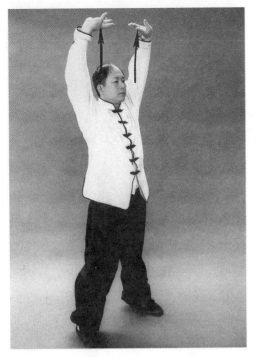

Figure 3-120.

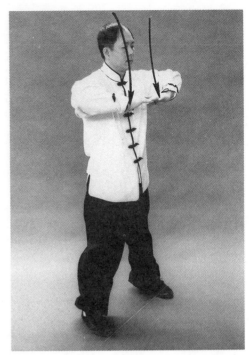

Figure 3-121.

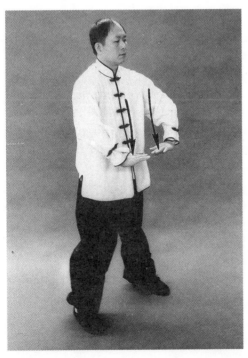

Figure 3-122.

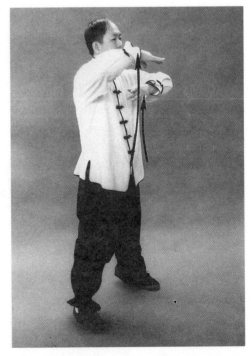

Figure 3-123.

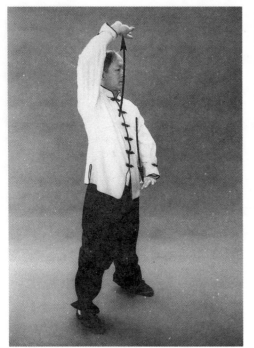

Figure 3-124.

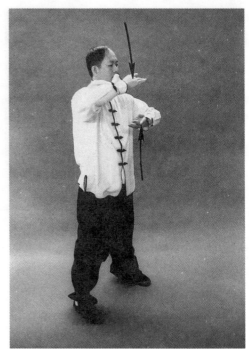

Figure 3-125.

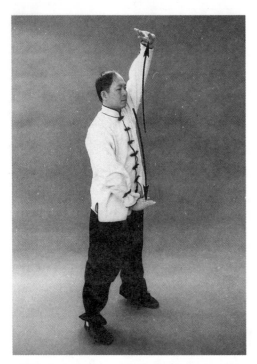

Figure 3-126.

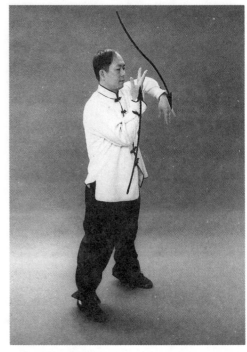

Figure 3-127.

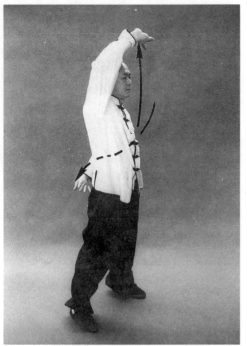

Figure 3-128.

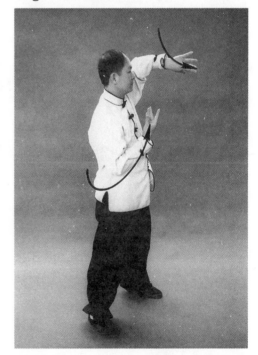

Figure 3-129.

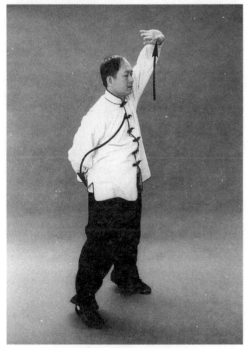

Figure 3-130.

Figure 3-131.

10. Turn your Head to Look at the Moon (Hwei Tour Wang Yeuh) 回頭望月

Continue from the last exercise with the same hand motion and breath coordination, but now twist your body as you exhale (Figures 3-131 and 3-132). When you inhale, twist your body to face the front and draw both hands to in front of your chest (Figure 3-133), and

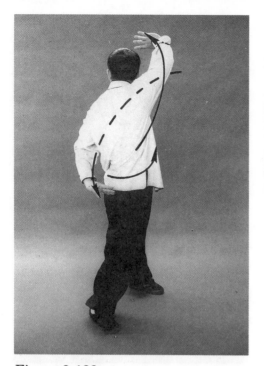

Figure 3-132.

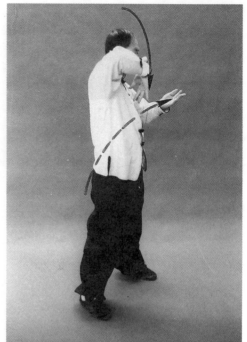

Figure 3-133.

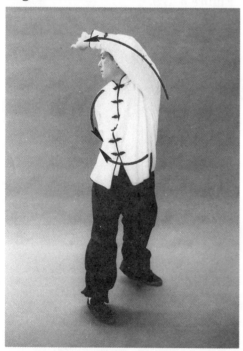

Figure 3-134.

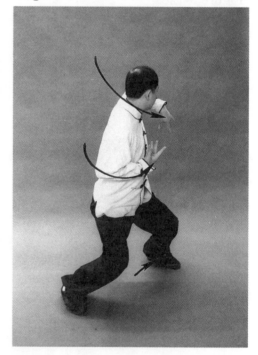

Figure 3-135.

when you exhale, twist your body to the side and separate your hands (Figure 3-134). If your right hand is up you should twist to the left, and vice versa. Repeat ten times.

11. Big Python Turns Its Body (Dah Maang Joan Shenn) 大蟒轉身

After you have finished the last exercise, step your left leg to the left and squat down to place about 60% of your weight on it. Your body twists and your arms move exactly as in the last exercise (Figures 3-135

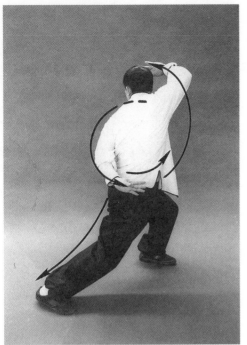

Figure 3-136.

Figure 3-137.

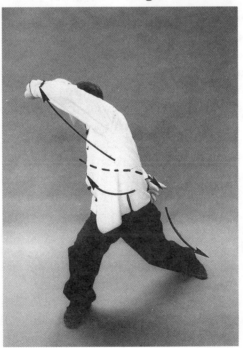

Figure 3-138.

and 3-136). When you twist your body to the left, also twist your head to look to your rear. Your right hand is above your head, and you are twisting your whole body from your fingertips to your feet. When you inhale, twist your body back to face forward while exchanging your hands (Figure 3-137). Finally, exhale and twist your body to the other side (Figure 3-138). Let your feet pivot as needed to keep your stance stable. Repeat the entire movement ten times.

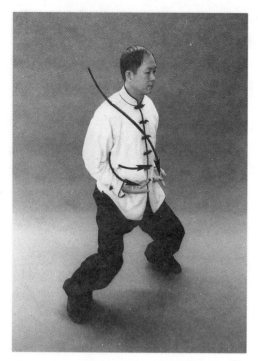 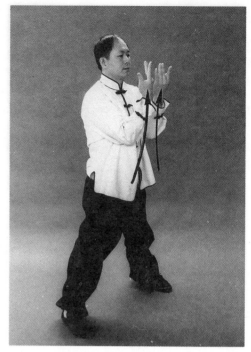

Figure 3-139.   Figure 3-140.

12. Up and Down Coiling (Shang Shiah Shyuan Parn) 上下旋盤

After you have completed the last exercise, turn your body to face forward and place your hands at your waist (Figure 3-139). Next, exhale and stand up, and at the same time raise your arms straight up with the palms facing forward (Figures 3-140 and 3-141). Then inhale and lower your body as you twist it to the rear, and simultaneously draw your arms in to your chest with the palms facing in. You should end up in the Sitting on Crossed Legs Stance (Figures 3-142 and 3-143). Then raise and twist your body to the front into the Horse Stance (Figure 3-144), and continue to raise your hands over your head, rotating the palms outward (Figure 3-145). Your feet should pivot as needed to keep your stance stable. Repeat the same movement to the other side (Figures 3-146 to 3-148). Repeat ten times. After you finish, inhale and bring the hands down to your chest (Figure 3-149), and then exhale and lower them down to your waist (Figure 3-150). The entire body is like a spring, bouncing and coiling up and down slowly in coordination with the breathing. Weak or older practitioners may find this exercise too strenuous. If this is the case, either skip it, or reduce the number of repetitions.

After you have finished the entire coiling set, stand still, and regulate your mind and breathing for a few minutes (Figure 3-151). Feel the Chi redistributing. Remain standing for a couple of minutes before you move.

III. Rocking Set

The rocking set was originally designed to teach the martial Tai Chi practitioner to balance his Chi when doing Jing. It says in Chang San-Feng's Treatise: "If there is a top, there is a bottom; if

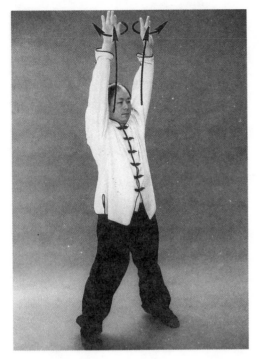

Figure 3-141.

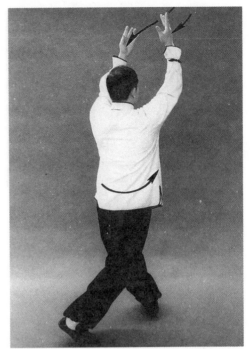

Figure 3-142.

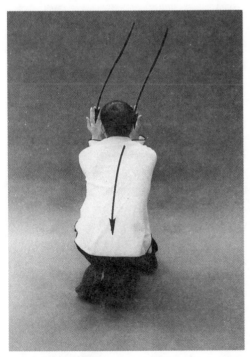

Figure 3-143.

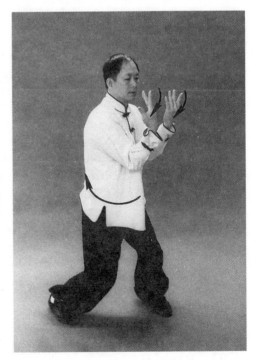

Figure 3-144.

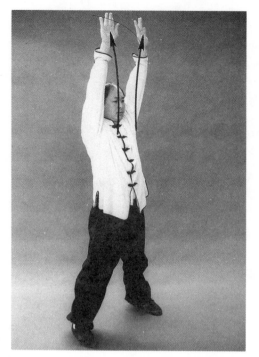

Figure 3-145.

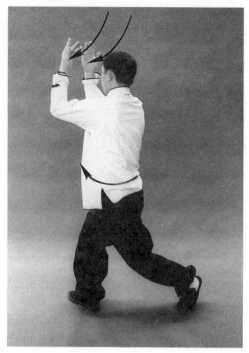

Figure 3-146.

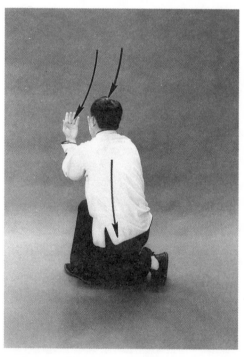

Figure 3-147.

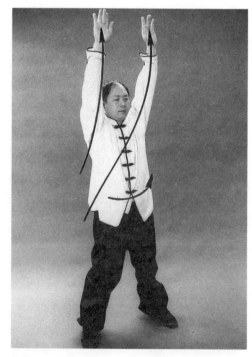

Figure 3-148.

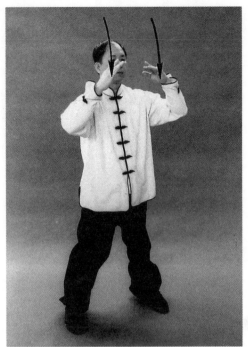
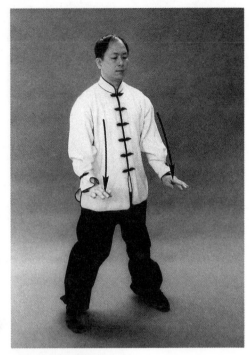

Figure 3-149.   Figure 3-150.

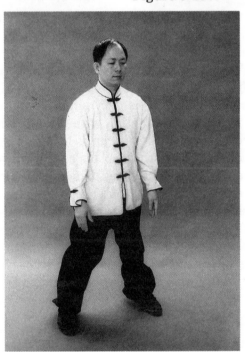

Figure 3-151.

there is a front, there is a back; if there is a left, there is a right. If Yi wants to go upward, this implies considering downward."(*3) From this saying it is very clear that the secret of effective Jing manifestation is balanced Yi and Chi.

(*3). 張三豐: ＂有上即有下，有前即有後，有左即
有右，如意要向上，即寓下意．＂

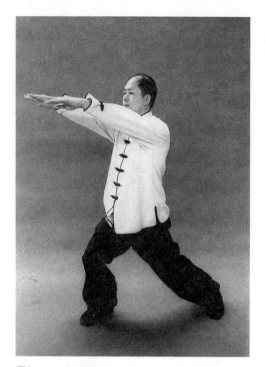 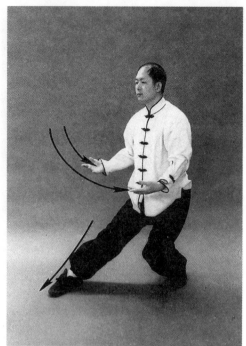

Figure 3-152.   Figure 3-153.

To analyze this subject further, Jing balance includes first balancing the posture, which comes from firm rooting and centering. Only then will the body be comfortable and stable, and the judgement of the Yi accurate. When this Yi is used to lead the Chi to energize the muscles, you will be able to manifest your strongest Jing.

The motion of the rocking is very simple. You simply shift your weight from leg to leg in coordination with the arm movements. When you move forward, the action of the arms is balanced by the rear leg, and when you shift your weight to the rear leg and withdraw your arms, the movement is balanced by the front leg. The repeated rocking movement helps you to develop a feeling for centering and balancing, and to build the root from which power can be grown. Although this set was originally created for Jing training, many Tai Chi practitioners have found that it can significantly improve leg strength and also train both physical and mental centering and balance. This also contributes to good health.

We will introduce only five exercises, but after you have practiced them for a while and understand the theory, you should be able to find or create others.

1.   Embracing Arms (Goong Bi) 拱臂

Start in the Bow and Arrow Stance, with 60% of your weight on your front foot and both arms stretched out in front of you (Figure 3-152). Inhale and shift your weight slowly back to your rear foot until it carries 60% of the weight. As you shift back, lower and draw in your arms while rotating them so that the palms are facing up (Figure 3-153). Continue to circle both arms sidewards and up to shoulder height. As you raise your arms, rotate them so that the palms are facing down when they reach shoulder height (Figure 3-

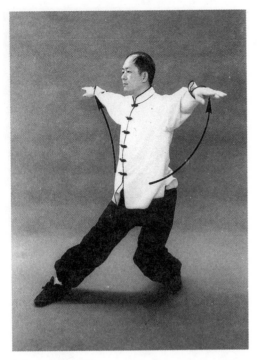 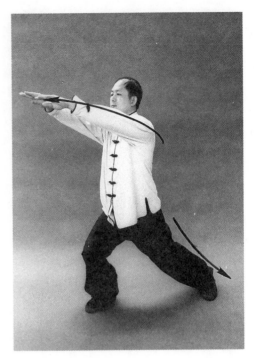

Figure 3-154.   Figure 3-155.

154). Then exhale and move both hands forward while once again shifting 60% of the body's weight to the front leg (Figure 3-155). Repeat ten times, then switch your legs and repeat the same movement another ten times.

2.   Wardoff (Peng) 掤

This form is adapted from the Tai Chi sequence. Start with your right leg forward, your right arm in front of your chest with the palm facing in, and your left hand just behind and below the right arm with the palm facing forward. The rear hand should not touch the front arm (Figure 3-156). As you shift your weight to your rear leg, inhale and move both hands down (Figure 3-157). Continuing the motion, exhale and shift your weight to the front leg while raising both arms in a wardoff movement (Figure 3-158). The motion is generated from the legs, and directed by the waist out to the right arm and left hand. Repeat the motion ten times, and then switch legs for another ten repetitions.

3.   Rollback and Press (Lu Ghi) 擺擠

This movement is also adapted from the Tai Chi form. Start in the right Bow and Arrow Stance with your right arm in front of your chest and your left hand behind the right wrist (Figure 3-159). Exhale and coil your right hand forward and upward like a snake coiling up a branch (Figures 3-160 and 3-161). Your left hand stays next to your right arm and follows its movements. As you inhale, smoothly continue the motion by turning your right palm down and starting the rollback movement while shifting your weight to the rear leg until you are in the Four-Six Stance and your body is turned

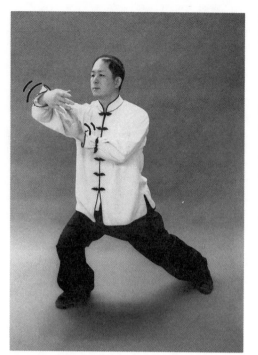

Figure 3-156.

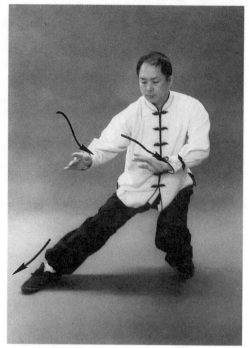

Figure 3-157.

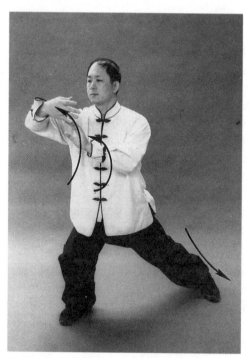

Figure 3-158.

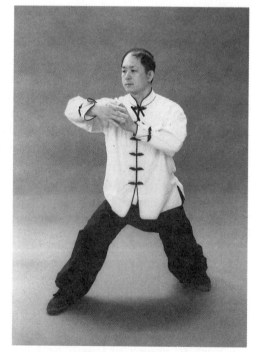

Figure 3-159.

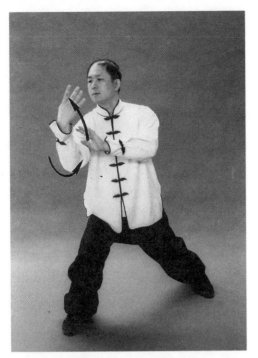

Figure 3-160.

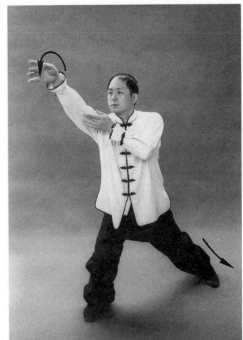

Figure 3-161.

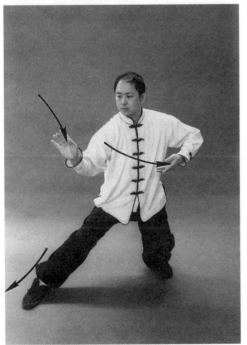

Figure 3-162.

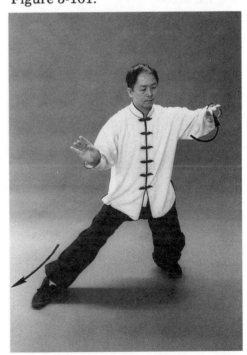

Figure 3-163.

slightly to the left (Figure 3-162). Move your left arm through a small circle (Figure 3-163), and then touch your left hand to your right wrist (Figure 3-164). Finally, exhale and use the left hand to press the right wrist forward as you shift 60% of your weight to the front leg (Figure 3-165). After you have finished ten repetitions, switch your legs and do ten repetitions on the other side.

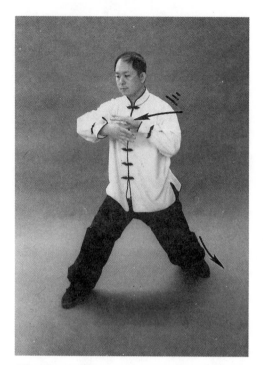

Figure 3-164.

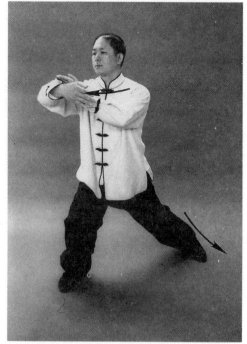

Figure 3-165.

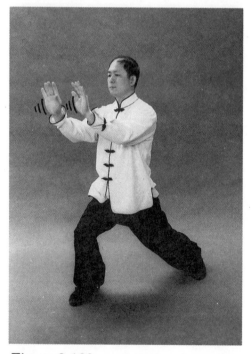

Figure 3-166.

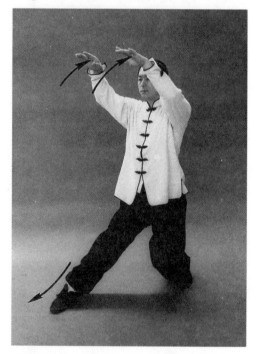

Figure 3-167.

4. Push (An) 按

This movement is also adapted from the Tai Chi sequence. Start by pushing forward with both hands while in the Bow and Arrow Stance (Figure 3-166). As you inhale, shift your weight to your rear leg into the Four-Six Stance, and simultaneously raise your hands up and then draw them back to your chest (Figures 3-167 and 3-168). As you

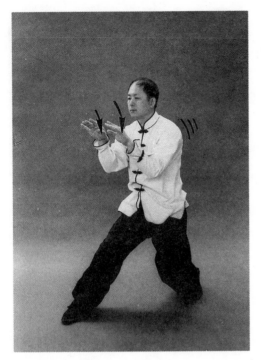 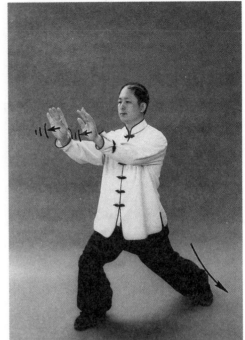

Figure 3-168.   Figure 3-169.

exhale, push your hands forward while once again shifting your weight forward into the Bow and Arrow Stance (Figure 3-169). When you push you should remain relaxed, but you should really feel that you are pushing a heavy object. Always remember: you must push your rear leg backward in order to obtain forward pushing power. Repeat ten times on each leg.

5.   Rotating the Ball (Joan Chyou) 轉球

Rotating the ball teaches the Tai Chi practitioner how to relax and soften the waist and chest, and also how to use the waist to direct the movements of the arms and hands. There is no specific pattern of movements in this exercise. You simply hold your arms in front of your chest with the palms facing each other as if you were holding a basketball, and then rotate the ball around in various ways and also move it up, down, and to the sides. You can turn your body in various directions, raise and lower it, and shift forward and backward (Figures 3-170 and 3-171). Generate the movement from your legs and direct it with your waist. You may rotate the ball any way you want as long as your palms remain facing each other and stay the same distance apart. Practice three minutes with the right leg forward and then change legs and practice for another three minutes.

You may have noticed that these exercises all work to develop the connection from the rooted legs to the waist, chest, shoulders, and finally to the hands. This is the most essential requirement in Tai Chi practice. In order to reach this goal your body must be very soft, and the movement from the legs to the hands must be continuous and without any stagnation. This builds a firm foundation for moving Tai Chi Chuan and also for manifesting Jing.

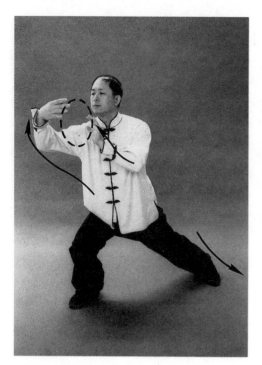

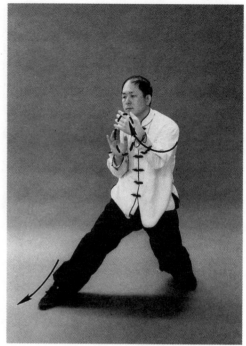

Figure 3-170.   Figure 3-171.

Walking Tai Chi Chi Kung

    Walking Tai Chi Chi Kung is essentially Tai Chi Chuan itself. Most of the walking movements are adapted from the Tai Chi sequence, the only difference being that a single movement is repeated continuously until you can feel the movement of Chi. Since you are only doing one basic movement it is easy to remember and master, and you can put all your attention on being relaxed, centered, and balanced, and thereby regulate your body. Then you can start regulating your breathing and mind, which is the key to leading your Chi. Walking Tai Chi Chi Kung should be trained before the beginner starts learning the Tai Chi sequence. Experienced practitioners often practice walking Tai Chi Chi Kung to penetrate to a deeper understanding of Chi, the mind, and the body.

1.   Wave Hands in Clouds (Yun Shoou)   雲手

    Squat down into the Horse Stance with your hands at waist height (Figure 3-172). Inhale and circle your right hand to in front of your left hand (Figure 3-173) and upward to chest level (Figure 3-174). Keeping your weight in the center, exhale and turn your body to the right. The hands naturally follow the turn of the body (Figure 3-175). Once your body is turned, inhale and press your right hand down and lift your left arm up to chest height while moving your left leg to the side of the right leg (Figure 3-176). Then exhale and turn your body to the left, letting your hands follow naturally along (Figure 3-177). Continue by stepping your right leg to the right as you switch your hands, and then turn to the right as you start shifting your weight to the right leg. Repeat as many times as you wish. The arms should be very light, and should float around like clouds.

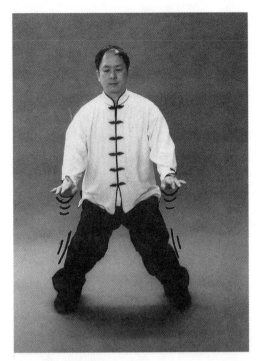

Figure 3-172.

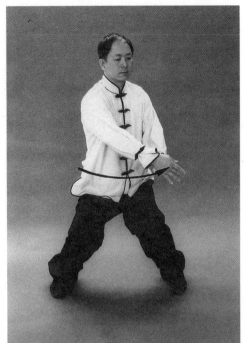

Figure 3-173.

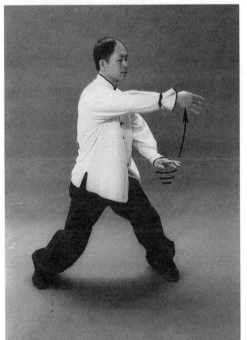

Figure 3-174.

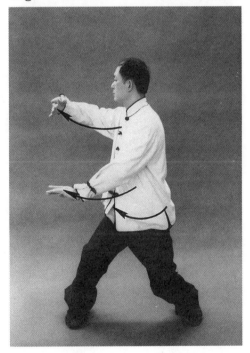

Figure 3-175.

The main purpose of this exercise is to loosen the waist and spine, and also to learn how to direct the power from the legs to the hands with a rotating motion.

2. Diagonal Flying (Xie Fei Shih) 斜飛勢

Start in the Bow and Arrow Stance with your left hand in front of your face and your right hand out to your side at lower

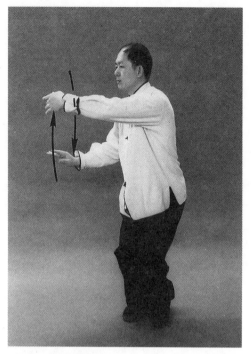

Figure 3-176.

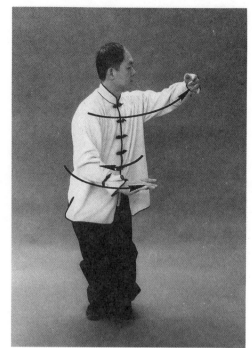

Figure 3-177.

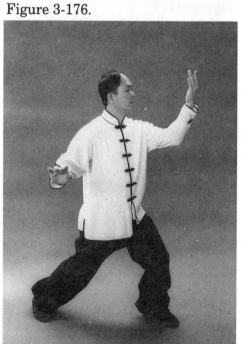

Figure 3-178.

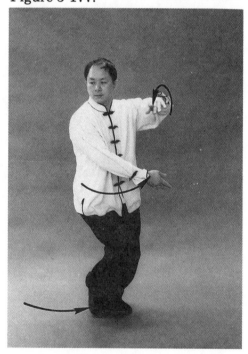

Figure 3-179.

chest height (Figure 3-178). As you inhale, rotate your body slightly to the left. As you turn, rotate your left arm so that the palm is facing down, pull your right arm in and rotate it so that the hand is palm up under the left hand, and also pull in your right leg next to your left leg (Figure 3-179). Step your right leg out to the right front. As you exhale, shift 60% of your weight forward onto your right leg, rotate your body toward the right leg,

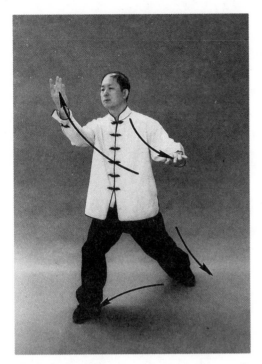 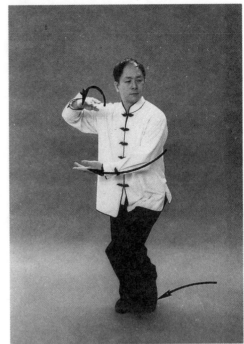

Figure 3-180.   Figure 3-181.

and separate your arms (Figure 3-180). The movement of the
right arm is powered by the rotation of the body. The right arm
should not go out past the side of the body. Next, inhale and
rotate your body slightly to your right. At the same time, rotate
your right arm so the palm faces down, draw in the left arm and
rotate it so that the hand is palm up under the right hand, and
draw in your left leg (Figure 3-181). Step your left leg out to your
left front, then exhale and shift your body forward. At the same
time, rotate your body toward the left leg and separate your arms
so that you end up in the position you started from. While practicing this movement you should arc in your chest as you inhale,
and expand it as you exhale. This exercise is very useful for regulating the Chi in the lungs and kidneys.

3.   Twist Body and Circle Fists (Pieh Shenn Chui) 撇身捶

Step your right leg forward and touch the heel down, and at the
same time move your right arm across your body (Figure 3-182). As
you exhale, shift your weight forward and twist your body so that
your foot turns to the right front and your right arm circles clockwise
in front of your chest (Figure 3-183). Your left arm moves with your
body. Inhale and step your left leg forward and touch the heel down,
and at the same time start lowering your right arm and moving your
left arm across your body. Then exhale and rotate your body to the
left so that your left foot turns to the left front and your left arm
circles counterclockwise up and to your left (Figure 3-184). Your
right arm moves with your body. Remember that the waist always
directs the movement of the arms. Practice at least ten times.

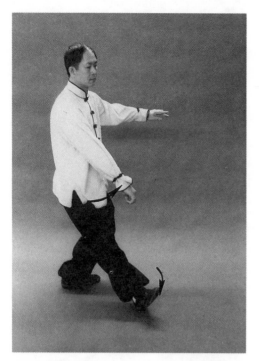

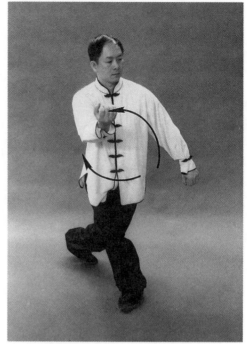

Figure 3-182.　　　　　　　　Figure 3-183.

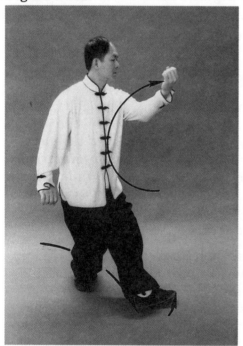

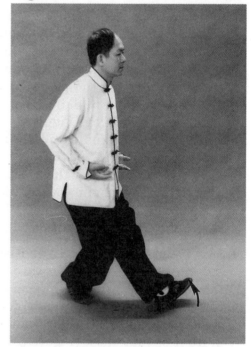

Figure 3-184.　　　　　　　　Figure 3-185.

4.　Stepping Leg (Tsai Tuei) 踩腿

Stepping leg is used to train balance and also to strengthen the knees. Inhale and step your left leg forward with the toes facing about 30 degrees to the left (Figure 3-185). Shift your weight to the left leg and at the same time slowly kick out with your right heel while pushing your left hand forward and exhaling

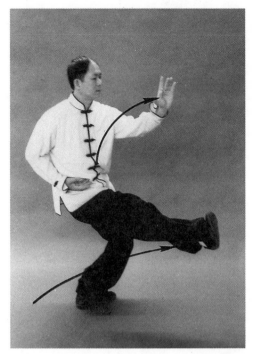

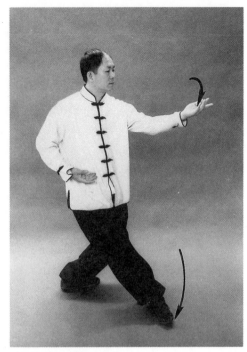

Figure 3-186.   Figure 3-187.

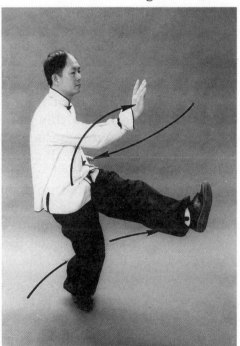

Figure 3-188.

(Figure 3-186). Inhale and step your right leg forward with the
toes pointing about 30 degrees to the right (Figure 3-187), and
then exhale and slowly kick the left leg out while pushing the
right hand forward (Figure 3-188). While you are pushing one
hand out, the other should pull back to your waist with the palm
facing upward. Practice ten times.

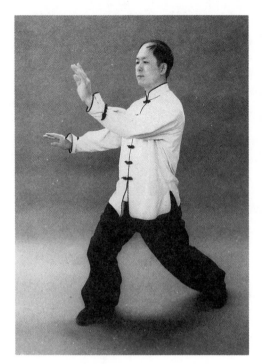 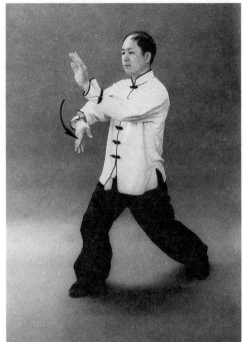

Figure 3-189.   Figure 3-190.

5.   Brush Knee and Step Forward (Lou Hsi Yao Bu) 摟膝拗步

Stand in the Bow and Arrow Stance with the right leg forward, your right hand at your waist, and your left hand pushing forward (Figure 3-189). Inhale and start to circle your right arm clockwise across your chest (Figure 3-190). As you exhale, rotate your body to the right, pivot your right foot to the right front corner, and push your left hand to your right. As you do this you are also shifting your weight to your front leg, and your right hand continues to circle down and to your right (Figure 3-191). Still exhaling, lift your left knee to waist height, circle your left arm down to brush past your knee, and circle your right arm back and up to by your right ear (Figure 3-192). Inhale and step your left leg forward (Figure 3-193). As you exhale, shift your weight forward, rotate your body to the front, push forward with your right hand, and draw your left arm back and down (Figure 3-194). Then repeat the entire sequence to the other side. Practice ten repetitions.

6.   Repulse Monkey (Dao Nien Hou) 倒撞猴

Start in the Four-Six Stance with your right leg forward, your right hand pushing forward, and your left hand at your waist (Figure 3-195). Next, inhale and rotate your right arm so the palm faces up, and at the same time circle your left hand back and up to behind your left ear while lifting your right leg up (Figure 3-196). Use the momentum of lifting your right leg to rotate your body and pivot on your left foot so that the toes face forward. Your left hand should reach the vicinity of your ear about this time (Figure 3-197). Then step your right leg back, exhale and shift your weight to the right leg, and at the same time push your left hand forward while withdrawing your right

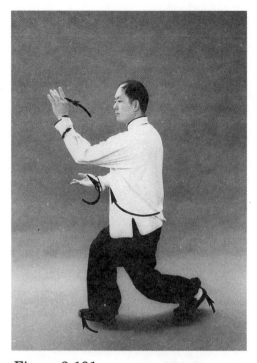

Figure 3-191.

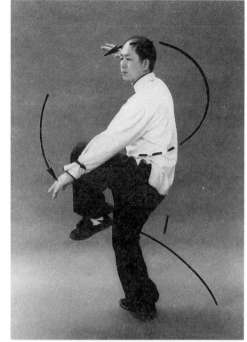

Figure 3-192.

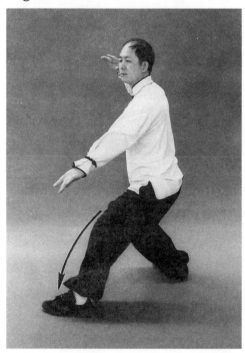

Figure 3-193.

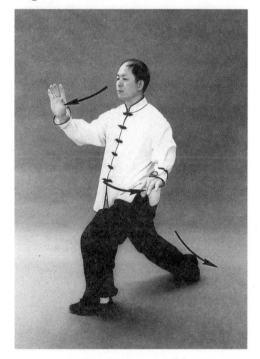

Figure 3-194.

hand back to your waist (Figure 3-198). Continue the same movement with the other leg and keep stepping backward ten times.

7. Snake Creeps Down (Sher Shenn Shiah Shih) 蛇身下勢
and Golden Rooster Stands on One Leg (Jin Ji Du Li) 金鷄獨立

Start in the Bow and Arrow Stance with the left palm pushing forward and the right hand raised behind you (the Single Whip

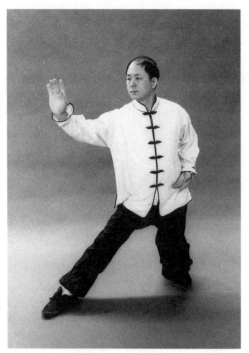

Figure 3-195.

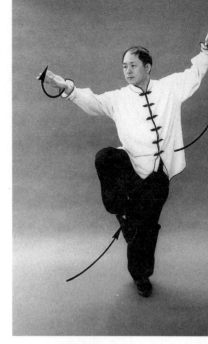

Figure 3-196.

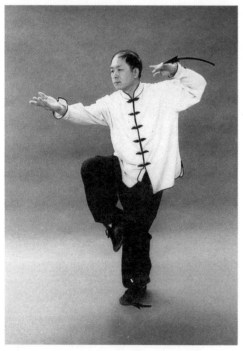

Figure 3-197.

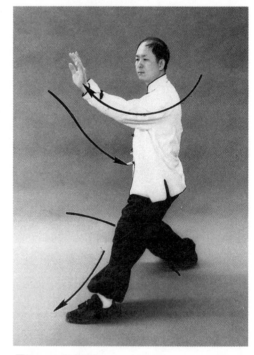

Figure 3-198.

posture)(Figure 3-199). As you inhale, shift your weight back to the right leg, squat down, and withdraw your left hand back to your chest (Figure 3-200). Circle your left hand down and move it along your left leg (Figure 3-201). Start to exhale, turn your left foot 30 degrees to the side while shifting your weight onto it. As your weight comes forward, first bend your knee and then straighten it partially. Your

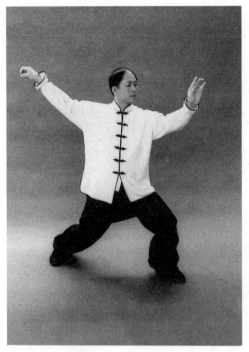

Figure 3-199.

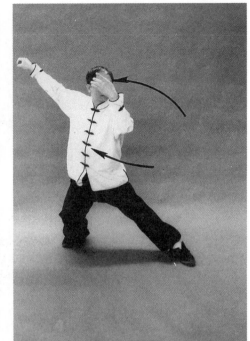

Figure 3-200.

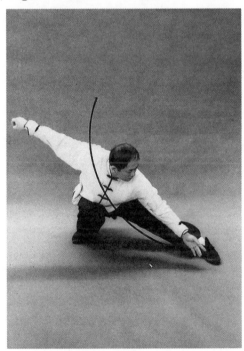

Figure 3-201.

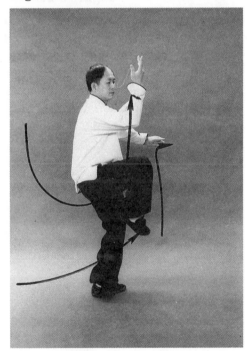

Figure 3-202.

right hand rises to in front of your face, your right knee rises to waist height, and your left hand moves to your left side (Figure 3-202). Finally, step your right leg forward, squat down, inhale and repeat the same movements on the other leg (Figure 3-203). Practice ten times.

When you train these walking Chi Kung exercises, the movements as always start from the legs, are directed by the waist, and

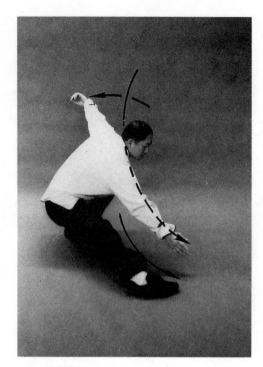

Figure 3-203.

finally reach to the hands. Practice until the movements are smooth and natural, the breathing is calm, deep, and comfortable, and your mind is meditatively concentrated. Remember to coordinate the movement of your Huiyin cavity and anus with your breathing. This is the key to advancing from external Tai Chi feeling into the field of internal Tai Chi sensing.

Chapter 4
Conclusion

There is so much to Tai Chi that it is impossible to cover all of its theory and training in only a few books. It is also impossible for anyone to claim that he thoroughly understands Tai Chi theory and has completed the training in his short lifetime. In fact, only those advanced Tai Chi players who have reached the essence of the art's theory and practice will understand its real depth. It seems that the more you dig, the deeper it is, and the more you open your eyes, the further you will see. We need many experienced Tai Chi masters to open their minds and share what they have learned with the public. Only in this way will the study of Tai Chi Chuan reach a profound level and benefit mankind.

I have had several goals in publishing this book. First, I hope to lead interested Tai Chi players into the field of the inner feelings of Tai Chi Chuan. Many people who practice Tai Chi Chuan today are only looking to relax their bodies, and they still pay most of their attention to regulating the physical body. I hope that through this book they will be able to access the inner side of Tai Chi practice. Second, I would like to help teach those who are interested in Tai Chi as a martial art the correct ways of moving the body, and also how to lead Chi to the limbs. A soft body and the coordination of the mind and Chi is the key to Tai Chi power. Tai Chi Chi Kung training will enable them to build the foundation for martial applications. Third, to introduce Tai Chi Chi Kung to those of the general public who would like to improve their health.

I hope that this book will generate wide effects, like a stone thrown in a pond. If this book can bring health to the general public, then my dream will have come true.

Appendix A
Glossary of Chinese Terms

Ann Mo: 按摩

Literally: press rub. Together they mean massage.

Ba Duann Gin: 八段錦

Eight Pieces of Brocade. A Wai Dan Chi Kung practice which is said to have been created by Marshal Yeuh Fei during the Song dynasty (1127-1279 A.D.).

Ba Kua: 八卦

Literally: Eight Divinations. Also called the Eight Trigrams. In Chinese philosophy, the eight basic variations; shown in the I Ching as groups of single and broken lines.

Ba Kua Chang: 八卦掌

Eight Trigrams Palm. One of the internal Chi Kung martial styles, believed to have been created by Doong Hae-Chuan between 1866 and 1880 A.D.

Bih Gang: 閉肛

Close the anus.

Chang Chuan: 長拳

Chang means long, and Chuan means fist, style, or sequence. A style of Northern Chinese Kung Fu which specializes in kicking and long range fighting. Chang Chuan has also been used to refer to Tai Chi Chuan.

Chang San-Feng: 張三豐

Said to have created Tai Chi Chuan in the Song dynasty (960-1279 A.D.), however there is no certain documentary proof of this.

Changqiang: 長強

Name of a cavity in the Governing Vessel, located in the tail-bone area.

Charn (Zen): 禪（忍）

A Chinese school of Mahayana Buddhism which asserts that enlightenment can be attained through meditation, self-contemplation, and intuition, rather than through study of scripture. Charn is called Zen in Japan.

Chen Jar Gou: 陳家溝

Name of the village of the Chen family, where Chen Style Tai Chi Chuan originated.

Chi: 氣

The general definition of Chi is: universal energy, including heat, light, and electromagnetic energy. A narrower definition of Chi refers to the energy circulating in human or animal bodies.

Chiaw Men: 竅門

Tricky or secret door. The trick or secret can lead the practitioner to the essence of the training.

Chii Huoo: 起火

To start the fire. In Chi Kung practice: when you start to build up Chi at the Lower Dan Tien.

Chi Kung: 氣功

Kung means Kung Fu (lit. energy-time). Therefore, Chi Kung means study, research, and/or practices related to Chi.

Chin Na: 擒拿

Literally, grab control. A type of Chinese Kung Fu which emphasizes grabbing techniques to control the opponent's joints in conjunction with attacking certain acupuncture cavities.

Ching: 經

Channel. Sometimes translated meridian. Refers to the twelve organ-related "rivers" which circulate Chi throughout the body.

Da Chyau: 搭橋

To build a bridge. Refers to the Chi Kung practice of touching the roof of the mouth with the tip of the tongue to form a bridge or link between the Governing and Conception Vessels.

Da Mo: 達摩

The Indian Buddhist monk who is credited with creating the Yi Gin Ching and Shii Soei Ching while at the Shaolin monastery. His last name was Sardili, and he was also known as Bodhidarma. He was formerly the prince of a small tribe in southern India.

Dan Diing Tao Kung: 丹鼎道功

The elixir cauldron way of Chi Kung. The Taoists' Chi Kung training.

Dan Tien: 丹田

Literally: Field of Elixir. Locations in the body which are able to store and generate Chi (elixir) in the body. The Upper, Middle, and Lower Dan Tiens are located respectively between the eyebrows, at the solar plexus, and a few inches below the navel.

Dien Shiuh: 點穴

Dien means "to point and exert pressure" and Shiuh means "the cavities." Dien Shiuh refers to those Chin Na techniques which specialize in attacking acupuncture cavities to immobilize or kill an opponent.

Dih: 地

The Earth. Earth, Heaven (Tian), and Man (Ren) are the "Three Natural Powers" (San Tsair).

Dih Chi: 地氣

Earth Chi. The energy of the earth.

Dih Lii Shy: 地理師

Dih Lii means geomancy and Shy means teacher. Therefore Dih Lii Shy means a teacher or master who analyzes geographic locations according to formulas in the I Ching (Book of Change) and the energy distributions in the Earth.

Dim Mak: 點脉

Pointing the Vessels. The way of striking Chi or blood vessels in Chinese martial arts. See also Dien Shiuh.

Ermei Mountain: 峨嵋山

A mountain located in Szechuan province in China. Many martial Chi Kung styles originated there.

Fa Jing: 發劲

Emitting Jing. The power which is usually used for an attack.

Faan Hu Shi: 反呼吸

Reverse Breathing. Also commonly called Taoist Breathing.

Faan Jieng Buu Nao: 返精補腦

Literally: to return the Essence to nourish the brain. A Taoist Chi Kung training process wherein Chi which has been converted from Essence is led to the head to nourish the brain.

Faan Torng: 返童

Back to childhood. A training in Nei Dan Chi Kung through which the practitioner tries to regain control of the muscles of the lower abdomen.

Fengfu: 風府

Cavity name. Belongs to the Governing Vessel, located on the back of the head.

Feng Shoei Shy: 風水師

Literally: wind water teacher. Teacher or master of geomancy. Geomancy is the art or science of analyzing the natural energy relationships in a location, especially the interrelationships between "wind" and "water," hence the name. Also called Dih Lii Shy.

Gin Jong Jaw: 金鐘罩

Golden Bell Cover. An Iron Shirt training.

Goe Chi: 鬼氣

The Chi residue of a dead person. It is believed by the Chinese Buddhists and Taoists that this Chi residue is a so called ghost.

Hou Tian Faa: 後天法

Post Heaven Techniques. An internal style of martial Chi Kung which is believed to have been created around the sixth century.

Hsin: 心

Literally: Heart. Refers to the emotional mind.

Hsing Yi or Hsing Yi Chuan: 形意，形意拳

Literally: Shape-mind Fist. An internal style of Kung Fu in which the mind or thinking determines the shape or movement of the body. Creation of the style attributed to Marshal Yeuh Fei.

Hsin Shyi Shiang Yi: 心息相依

The emotional mind and breathing mutually relying on each other. A method of regulating the mind in Chi Kung in which the practitioner pays attention to his breathing in order to clear his mind of disturbance.

Hwang Tyng: 黄庭

Yellow yard. 1. A yard or hall in which Taoists, who often wore yellow robes, meditate together. 2. In Chi Kung training, a spot in the abdomen where it is believed that you are able to generate an "embryo."

I Ching: 易經

Book of Changes. A book of divination written during the Jou dynasty (1122-255 B.C.).

Jargi: 夾脊

A cavity name used by Chi Kung practitioners. The acupuncture name for the same cavity is Lingtai. This cavity in on the Governing Vessel. See also Lingtai.

Jea Guu Wen: 甲骨文

Oracle-Bone Scripture. Earliest evidence of the Chinese use of the written word. Found on pieces of turtle shell and animal bone from the Shang dynasty (1766-1154 B.C.). Most of the information recorded was of a religious nature.

Jeng Hu Shi: 正呼吸

Normal Breathing. More commonly called Buddhist Breathing.

Jieng: 精

Essence. The most refined part of anything.

Jieng Tzu: 精子

Sons of the essence. Refers to the sperm.

Jing: 勁

A power in Chinese martial arts which is derived from muscles which have been energized by Chi to their maximum potential.

Kan: 坎

A phase of the eight trigrams representing water.

Kung Fu: 功夫

Literally: energy-time. Any study, learning, or practice which requires a lot of patience, energy, and time to complete. Since practicing Chinese martial arts requires a great deal of time and energy, Chinese martial arts are commonly called Kung Fu.

Kuoshu: 國術

Literally: national techniques. Another name for Chinese martial arts. First used by President Chiang Kai-Shek in 1926 at the founding of the Nanking Central Kuoshu Institute.

Laogong: 勞宮

Cavity name. On the Pericardium channel in the center of the palm.

Lao Tzyy: 老子

The creator of Taoism, also called Li Erh.

Li: 力

The power which is generated from muscular strength.

Li Erh: 李耳

Lao Tzyy, the creator of Taoism.

Liann Chi: 練氣

Liann means to train, to strengthen, and to refine. A Taoist training process through which your Chi grows stronger and more abundant.

Lii: 離

A phase of the Ba Kua, Lii represents fire.

Lingtai: 靈臺

Spiritual station. In acupuncture, a cavity on the back. In Chi Kung, it refers to the Upper Dan Tien.

Liu Ho Ba Fa: 六合八法

Literally: six combinations eight methods. A style of Chinese internal martial arts reportedly created by Chen Bor during the Song dynasty (960-1279 A.D.).

Lou: 絡

The small Chi channels which branch out from the primary Chi channels and are connected to the skin and to the bone marrow.

Mei: 脉

Chi vessels. The eight vessels involved with transporting, storing, and regulating Chi.

Mih Tzong Shen Kung: 密宗神功

Secret Style of Spiritual Kung Fu. Tibetan Chi Kung and martial arts.

Nei Dan: 內丹

Internal elixir. A form of Chi Kung in which Chi (the elixir) is built up in the body and spread out to the limbs.

Nei Jing: 內勁

Internal Power. The Jing or power in which Chi from the Dan Tien is used to support the muscles. This is characterized by relatively relaxed muscles. When the muscles predominate and local Chi is used to support them, it is called Wai Jing. See also Wai Jing.

Nei Kung: 內功

Internal Kung Fu. The Chinese martial styles which emphasize building up Chi internally in the beginning, and later use this Chi to energize the muscles to a higher degree of efficiency. See also Wai Kung.

Nei Shyh Kung Fu: 內視功夫

Nei Shyh means to look internally, so Nei Shyh Kung Fu refers to the art of looking inside yourself to read the state of your health and the condition of your Chi.

Pai Huo: 白鶴

White Crane. A style of southern Shaolin Kung Fu which imitates the fighting techniques of the crane.

Ren Mei: 任脉

Usually translated "Conception Vessel."

Ren Chi: 人氣

Human Chi.

Ru Jia: 儒家

Literally: Confucian family. Scholars following the ideas of Confucian thoughts; Confucianists.

San Bao: 三寶

Three treasures. Essence (Jieng), energy (Chi), and spirit (Shen). Also called San Yuan (three origins).

San Guan: 三關

Three gates. In Small Circulation training, the three cavities on the Governing Vessel which are usually obstructed and must be opened.

Sann Kung: 散功

Energy dispersion. Premature degeneration of the muscles when the Chi cannot effectively energize them. Caused by earlier overtraining.

San Shih Chi Shih: 三十七勢

Thirty-Seven Postures. According to historical records, one of the predecessors of Tai Chi Chuan.

San Tsair: 三才

Three powers. Heaven, Earth, and Man.

Shaolin: 少林

A Buddhist temple in Henan province, famous for its martial arts.

Sheau Jeau Tian: 小九天

·Small nine heaven. A Chi Kung style created in the sixth century.

Sheau Jou Tian: 小周天

Small heavenly cycle. Also called Small Circulation. The completed Chi circuit through the Conception and Governing Vessels.

Shen: 神

Spirit. Said to reside in the Upper Dan Tien (the third eye).

Shenn Hsin Pyng Herng: 身心平衡

The body and the mind are mutually balanced. In Chinese Chi Kung, the physical body is Yang and the mind is Yin. They must both be trained to balance each other.

Shen Shyi Shiang Yi: 神息相依

The Shen and breathing mutually rely on each other. A stage in Chi Kung practice.

Shian Tian Chi: 先天氣

Pre-birth Chi. Also called Dan Tien Chi. The Chi which was converted from Original Essence and is stored in the Lower Dan Tien. Considered to be "Water Chi," it is able to calm the body.

Shii Soei Ching: 洗髓經

Washing Marrow/Brain Classic, usually translated Marrow/Brain Washing Classic. Chi Kung training specializing in leading Chi to the marrow to cleanse it.

Shiou Chi: 修氣

Cultivate the Chi. Cultivate implies to protect, maintain, and refine. A Buddhist Chi Kung training.

Shoou Jing: 守勁

Defensive Jing. The Jings which are used for defense.

Suann Ming Shy: 算命師

Literally: calculate life teacher. A fortune teller who is able to calculate your future and destiny.

Tai Chi Chuan: 太极拳

Great ultimate fist. An internal martial art.

Tao: 道

The way. The "natural" way of everything.

Tao Jia (Tao Jiaw): 道家（道教）

The Tao family. Taoism. Created by Lao Tzyy during the Jou dynasty (1122-934 B.C.). In the Han dynasty (c. 58 A.D.), it was mixed with Buddhism to become the Taoist religion (Tao Jiaw).

Tao Te Ching: 道德經

Morality Classic. Written by Lao Tzyy.

Tian Chi: 天氣

Heaven Chi. It is now commonly used to mean the weather, since weather is governed by heaven Chi.

Tian Chyr: 天池

Heavenly pond. The place under the tongue where saliva is generated.

Tian Shyr: 天時

Heavenly timing. The repeated natural cycles generated by the heavens such as the seasons, months, days, and hours.

Tiea Bu Shan: 鐵布衫

Iron shirt. Kung Fu training which toughens the body externally and internally.

Tuei Na: 推拿

Literally: push and grab. A style of massage and manipulation for treatment of injuries and many illnesses.

Tyau Chi: 嗣氣

To regulate the Chi.

Tyau Hsin: 嗣心

To regulate the emotional mind.

Tyau Shen: 嗣神

To regulate the spirit.

Tyau Shenn: 嗣身

To regulate the body.

Tyau Shyi: 嗣息

To regulate the breathing.

Wai Dan: 外丹

External elixir. External Chi Kung exercises in which Chi is built up in the limbs and then led to the body.

Wai Jing: 外勁

External Power. The type of Jing where the muscles predominate and only local Chi is used to support the muscles. See also Nei Jing.

Wai Kung: 外功

External Kung Fu. The Chinese martial styles which emphasize mainly muscular power and strength in the beginning. See also Nei Kung.

Wey Chi: 衛氣

Guardian Chi. The Chi shield which wards off negative external influences.

Weilu: 尾閭

Tailbone. The name used by Chinese martial artists and Chi Kung practitioners. The acupuncture name for this cavity is Changqiang. See also Changqiang.

Woa Shoou: 瓦手

Tile Hand. The typical open-hand form used in Tai Chi Chuan.

Wu Chi: 無极

No Extremity. This is the state of undifferentiated emptiness before a beginning. As soon as there is a beginning or a movement, there is differentiation and opposites, and this is called Tai Chi.

Wushu: 武術

Literally: martial techniques. A common name for the Chinese martial arts. Many other terms are used, including: Wuyi (martial arts), Wukung (martial Kung Fu), Kuoshu (national techniques), and Kung Fu (energy-time). Because Wushu has been modified in mainland China over the past forty years into gymnastic martial performance, many traditional Chinese martial artist have given up this name in order to avoid confusing modern Wushu with traditional Wushu. Recently, mainland China has attempted to bring modern Wushu back toward its traditional training and practice.

Wuudang Mountain: 武當山

Located in Fubei province in China.

Yang: 陽

In Chinese philosophy, the active, positive, masculine polarity. In Chinese medicine, Yang means excessive, overactive, overheated. The Yang (or outer) organs are the Gall Bladder, Small Intestine, Large Intestine, Stomach, Bladder, and Triple Burner.

Yeuh Fei: 岳飛

A Chinese hero in the Southern Song dynasty (1127-1279 A.D.). Said to have created Ba Duann Gin, Hsing-Yi Chuan, and Yeuh's Ien Jao.

Yi: 意

Mind. Specifically, the mind which is generated by clear thinking and judgement, and which is able to make you calm, peaceful, and wise.

Yi Gin Ching: 易筋經

Literally: changing muscle/tendon classic, usually called The Muscle/Tendon Changing Classic. Credited to Da Mo around 550 A.D., this work discusses Wai Dan Chi Kung training for strengthening the physical body.

Yi Shoou Dan Tien: 意守丹田

Keep your Yi on your Dan Tien. In Chi Kung training, you keep your mind at the Dan Tien in order to build up Chi. When you are circulating your Chi, you always lead your Chi back to your Dan Tien before you stop.

Yii Yi Yiin Chi: 以意引氣

Use your Yi (wisdom mind) to lead your Chi. A Chi Kung technique. Chi cannot be pushed, but it can be led. This is best done with the Yi.

Yin: 陰

In Chinese philosophy, the passive, negative, feminine polarity. In Chinese medicine, Yin means deficient. The Yin (internal) organs are the Heart, Lungs, Liver, Kidneys, Spleen, and Pericardium.

Ying Chi: 營氣

Managing Chi. It manages the functioning of the organs and the body.

Ying Kung: 硬功

Hard Kung Fu. The Chinese martial styles which emphasize hard Jing training.

Yuan Chi: 元氣

Original Chi. The Chi created from the Original Essence inherited from your parents.

Yuan Jieng: 元精

Original Essence. The fundamental, original substance inherited from your parents, it is converted into Original Chi.

Yuhjeen: 玉枕

Jade pillow. One of the three gates of Small Circulation training.